For This Child I Prayed:
A Journey of Hope and Healing

Clair Chandler Rivera

For This Child I Prayed: A Journey of Hope and Healing

Back cover photo courtesy of Amy Pennington Photography.

Library of Congress Cataloging-in-Publication Data

Rivera, Clair Chandler, 1975-.
        For this child I prayed: a journey of hope and healing / Clair
Chandler Rivera -- First Edition. All rights reserved.
ISBN 978-0-578-05687-6

Printed in the United States of America

Table of Contents

Acknowledgments

First and foremost, my Lord and Savior, Jesus Christ. Thank you, Lord, for seeing more in me than anyone else ever has or will, and for the glorious freedom that comes only from being your child. I owe everything I am and will ever become solely to you. *Hear the song of my life. Let it be a sweet, sweet sound.*

My incredible husband and best friend, Victor. I could never have completed this project without your support, input and countless hours of review. Our marriage is proof that "happily ever after" isn't limited to fairy tales. You are a precious gift and an answer to prayer. You're everything I ever wanted in a lifelong partner, and then some. I fall more in love with you every day.

Ryan and Brooklyn – my precious angel babies. I look at you every day with complete awe, wonder, and pride that I have the privilege of being your mommy. I wanted each of you so much and prayed for you for so long that it is still surreal to finally have you here in my arms. Everything I want to say and teach you boils down to this: love Jesus above all else, seek Him in everything you do, and He will take care of you far better than I ever could.

Elmer and Darlene – my parents. Thank you for making Jesus a priority in our family, for teaching me His ways and doing your absolute best to make sure I stayed on the narrow path. Now that I am an adult, thank you for becoming some of my closest friends.

"Rachel" – the woman who gave birth to me. Thank you for choosing life and for allowing me to be part of yours.

"Valerie" – Ryan's birthmother. You will always have a special place in our hearts, and we thank God every day for you. Thank you so much for our little man. He is an absolute joy and a precious gift.

Kelly Lively King – my best friend. You are such an inspiration and a blessing. Thank you for believing in me and being that friend that "sticks closer than a brother" (and for teaching me that all of life's major issues can be solved over Starbucks drinks and/or consuming large quantities of chocolate). I love you so much.

Jennifer Selman – my "favorite friend." Our friendship has endured so much and I am so glad that I didn't lose you in the process. I love you.

Our spiritual leaders and pastors, Mike and LaNell Martindale at The Heights Fellowship in Lubbock, Texas; Tommy and Donna Politz at Hillside Christian Church in Amarillo, Texas; and Bill and Cindy Ramsey at The Met Church in Keller, Texas.

My friend and co-editor, Sarah Broad. Your encouragement, friendship, and prayer have been invaluable. God bless you.

Those who stayed the course with us through the ups and downs of this journey: Chad and Debbie Padgett, Judy Stallwitz, Randi Gutierrez, Janis Alexander Cross, Darla Lynn, Walt Weaver, Cindy Gilliland, Carissa Wingate, and Geeta Yadav Singletary.

Introduction

The confused stare was one my husband, Victor, and I had grown accustomed to. The woman locked her gaze on us and quickly headed our direction. *Here we go again.* I took a deep breath and forced a smile, though admittedly not an entirely sincere one.

"How old is he?" She smiled as knelt in front of the stroller.

"Four months."

Wait for it. There it is - the look of bewilderment and disbelief as she stared at my round belly, the nubbin of my bellybutton protruding ever so slightly beneath the stretchy material of my shirt. I could see the wheels turning in her head as she tried to quickly and tactfully determine if I was smuggling a melon, pregnant or just fat.

"And when are you due?" This was my favorite part.

"Next week," I smiled sweetly.

I normally took the time to at least explain the abbreviated version of how our little family came to be, but not today. This was far too entertaining to give in so easily.

Before the baffled stranger could say another word, the restaurant hostess called our name. Perfect timing. As we walked away, I glanced over my shoulder at the woman, who continued to stare at me with a mixture of wonder and horror as if I had suddenly sprouted a third eye.

I have told the short version of our story countless times but it does not even begin to scratch the surface. I am now sharing my journey and ultimately my heart in its barest form,

1

earnestly praying that it will somehow offer hope and encouragement to women who have struggled with infertility, miscarriage, or who have given a child up for adoption.

Every woman who has been down one of these roads has a unique story that makes the experience personal to her, yet we are bound together by a common tapestry of emotions we can all relate to: loss, disappointment, jealousy, bitterness, desperation, grief, rejection, hopelessness, isolation, anger, guilt, depression...just to name a few. If this is you, then you're in good company.

If you are anything like I was, you feel like no one truly understands what you're going through or the depth of your pain. You don't want to hear another statistic about how many couples experience infertility or how many pregnancies end in miscarriage. If you have made the most selfless decision I can think of and placed a baby for adoption, you don't want to hear that the baby is better off; or worse, have one more person judge or criticize your decision.

You don't want anyone to hug you (especially when it is preceded with "the sympathy look") because you have avoided any form of a melt-down for the last three hours, breaking a personal record. You are a little miffed at the insensitive scrap who sent you the baby announcement or shower invitation. At the same time, you feel a stinging twinge of guilt for not being able to join in another woman's happiness.

You may be thinking, "What is *wrong* with me?" or wondering why you can't seem to snap out of it. You may have asked God, "Why *her* and not *me*?" or you may be so angry at

God that you have stopped talking to Him altogether. If any of this sounds remotely familiar, this book was written for you.

When I had my miscarriages, there were wonderful resources available on both physical and emotional healing, but nothing in regard to spiritual healing. I spent too many years believing God either did not hear my prayers or did not care. That in itself was very hard to admit to myself, much less to anyone else. I wish someone who had traveled this road before me could have taken my hand and walked me through it - just so I would know I was not alone - then pointed me in the right direction toward healing the deep wounds in my spirit.

My motivation in writing this book is found in 2 Corinthians 1:3-4: *God is our merciful Father and the source of all comfort. He comforts us in all our troubles so that we can comfort others. When they are troubled, we will be able to give them the same comfort God has given us.* I firmly believe God never wastes a hurt. If He can use what I have been through to help someone else heal, the pain was worth it.

It has been a very long and difficult journey to get to where I am now, but I am so grateful for it. I have learned so much about the person and character of Jesus along the way. His ways are truly much higher than mine (Isaiah 55:9). This is really *His* story. I simply have the privilege of putting it on paper. May He be glorified in what I am about to share.

Surely it was for my benefit that I suffered such anguish.
In your love you kept me from the pit of destruction;
You have put all my sins behind your back
(Isaiah 38:17, NIV).

Part I: When Hope Leads to Heartache

Hope deferred makes the heart sick... (Proverbs 13:12).

The Lord is close to the brokenhearted;
he rescues those whose spirits are crushed
(Psalm 34:18).

I am worn out waiting for your rescue,
But I have put my hope in your word.
My eyes are straining to see your promises come true.
When will you comfort me?
(Psalm 119:81-82).

Chapter 1: Empty Womb, Empty Heart

Rachel

The closet in the corner bedroom had become Rachel's*
safe place, her refuge. It was cramped and bore the musty smell
of moth balls, but the overcoats, sweaters and blankets muffled
her cries. At least she hoped so. The closet was the only place
she felt safe to pour out the floodgate of emotions she kept
bottled up during the day. She had cried herself to sleep in here
more times than she cared to remember, processing the chain of
events that had led her to this town, these people, and this
house.

Despite what Rachel's classmates had said behind her
back, she really was a nice girl - a nice girl who had gotten
caught up in the whirlwind of first love. She had met Brad* not
even a year ago, during the fall of her freshman year at a private
Christian college tucked away in a small, quaint town in
Oklahoma.

Rachel came from a broken home where no one ever
really understood or listened to her. And then she met Brad. He
was funny, charming, and easy to talk to. He soon became her
best friend. She gave him her heart. He gave her hope in return.
He said he loved her and promised to marry her; that if she truly
loved him, she would trust him. It would be alright to let down
her guard just this once. They were going to be married someday
anyway, right? But just once, during that momentary lapse of
judgment in the heat of passion, is all it took.

---

* Name has been changed to protect privacy.

When the doctor confirmed their greatest fear, that Rachel was indeed pregnant, Brad held her tight and stroked her long, brown hair as she cried. He promised to marry her right away. He just needed the weekend to go home and tell his parents what was going on. Brad told her not to worry, that his family would love her as much as he did, and that the wedding details would be worked out when he got back.

Rachel wore a path in the dingy dorm room carpet, pacing up and down that Sunday afternoon, running to the window every time she heard a car door slam. Just as she was about to be sick with nervousness and anticipation, she saw Brad's car pull to the curb. She bolted out the door, ready to feel safe in his arms. But once she saw his face, she knew something was different.

"You O.K.?" she asked.

Brad gazed straight ahead as if mesmerized by the road in front of him. He took a deep breath in through his nose, mouth tightly clamped, and raised one eyebrow ever so slightly before breaking an eternity of silence.

"Yeah, great. It's just that..."

The complete lack of inflection in his voice sent chills down her spine.

"Just that *what*?"

Brad reached up to rub the back of his neck, continuing to avoid direct eye contact.

"It's just that there are so many things I want to accomplish before having a family."

Her hands begin to shake and a cold sweat broke out across her forehead. He reached out to touch her knee but she instantly recoiled as if his fingers were venomous serpents.

"Have you, uh, thought about an abortion?" He paused to clear his throat. "I mean, it really is the best option. We could go on with our lives, forget this ever happened, finish college and get married when we're *ready* rather than being forced into it right now."

By now her bottom lip was quivering and she was blinded by an ocean of hot, salty tears that she tried to brush away with the back of her hand. This had to be a dream – a *nightmare* at that. What was happening?

Her mouth felt as if it were stuffed full of cotton balls as she tried to speak.

"I'm sorry. I don't think I heard you correctly. Did you say 'abortion'?"

"I know it sounds horrible, Rachel, but it will be O.K.," he said. "God understands where we're coming from and despite what you think right now, He *will* forgive us."

He paused a moment. "Look, my parents have offered to pay for it and arrange everything for us."

She couldn't believe what she was hearing. *Roe v. Wade* had just made national headlines legalizing abortion, but the idea was quickly pushed from her mind. Two wrongs don't make a right.

Who *was* this person next to her? The love of her life, the father of her baby, the one she thought she knew better than anyone in this world was suddenly a total stranger. She did not know him at all. She was already living with the gut wrenching

7

effects of one sin and was not anxious to willingly jump into another.

The more Brad pressured her, the more Rachel stood her ground. She told him she was having this baby with or without him, hoping, of course, that he would say she was right and that they should just go on with their original plan – getting married and weathering this storm together, for better, for worse.

Brad's hand, once again resting on her knee, now gripped the steering wheel so tightly she could see his knuckles turning a pale white. The longer they sat in silence, the more she realized she was going to be on her own.

He kissed her on the cheek when he dropped her off and told her he would call her later. But he didn't. He never called again. When she tried to talk to him, to find out what she had done wrong or what had made him grow so cold, he brushed her off, refusing to even make eye contact with her.

Word soon got out and Rachel felt like Hester Prynne in *The Scarlet Letter* on the small, Christian campus. Friends who once greeted her with smiles now turned their backs, as if they were afraid the dirtiness of her "sin" would rub off on them.

The other girls were cruel, acting as self-appointed judges and jury in order to mask their own insecurities. Like vultures, they gathered in dorm rooms and picked her apart with their words. "We really need to pray for Sister Rachel. I guess you've heard…" With gasps and mouths covered in shock and false sympathy, girls who had once been Rachel's friends now flipped through mental Rolodexes to see who else they could share this "prayer request" with.

These girls had their own skeletons in the closet. Secret sins they desperately tried to hide so that no one would see the innermost chambers of their hearts. But at least they didn't do *that*. Their own offenses were surely just misdemeanors in God's eyes while Rachel's was a felony, punishable by ostracism and disapproval.

Just like the woman caught in adultery, there was no loving concern for Rachel's welfare. No compassion or mercy. Church leaders and ministers stood with rocks in hand, towering over her in all of their piety, ready to stone the life out of her. She was called into the Dean's office for a private meeting, where he suggested that she find a more suitable place for a girl in her "predicament." She had broken the moral code and must now pay the consequences.

Rachel reluctantly told her father and stepmother that she was pregnant and that there would be no wedding as she had been promised. As expected, the conversation did not go well. Ugly words were exchanged. Her request to move home was adamantly denied. Instead, her father sarcastically suggested she could always go on welfare, a word that had always been uttered with disdain in their household. The family never had much but they earned what they *did* have through hard, honest work. Her father did not think highly of anyone who relied on the government for support. "*Those* people" were leaches, unworthy of respect or dignity.

Rachel had been rejected by the love of her life, family, friends, the school and her church. She had endured many lectures but received no compassion. She had no job and nowhere to go.   There was only one person in the world she had left to confide in who may be able to help her.

Professor Graham* always had a welcoming smile and a twinkle in his eyes like he knew a wonderful secret. He was everything Rachel had wished for in a father figure. He and his wife, Fiona*, sponsored a ministry team that she was a part of, and had taken her under their wing. "Prof" would be so disappointed in her, a thought she almost could not bear, but she had no other option. He was her only hope of kindness and wisdom in this, the darkest hour of her young life.

Rachel was met with the overwhelming odor of old library books mixed with Pine Sol as she opened the front door of the administration building. She quickly placed a hand over her mouth to keep from retching. Her heart pounded so loudly she feared the entire first floor of faculty and secretaries could hear it. She ducked her head, trying to ignore the stares and whispers, and walked briskly down the hall to the fourth office on the left.

Prof was seated at his desk and barely had a chance to look up before she collapsed in a wing back chair across from him and began to cry. Humiliating as it was, she told him everything: the pregnancy, Brad's suggestion of abortion, the judgmental stares and cruel shunning, her heartfelt longing to keep the baby but having nowhere to go, nowhere to turn and no idea what to do next.

Rachel braced herself for another lecture, but received understanding and grace instead. She looked up into Prof's eyes and knew that he was heartbroken for her. He prayed with her, asking the Lord for clear direction and leading during this difficult time.

Prof made a phone call to some friends of his, Elmer and Mary Ann Chandler, who lived in Texas. He trusted the Chandlers so much that they had been appointed guardians of his own two daughters if something were to happen to him and his wife. The Chandlers immediately agreed to take her into their home. Rachel would be away from this place, with its memories and heartaches, and could carefully make a decision about her future there.

Rachel felt welcomed in the Chandlers' home right away. Mary Ann and Elmer had always wanted children – a whole house full of them – but it had not happened the way they hoped. Mary Ann had contracted the measles during a pregnancy. The baby boy was stillborn and Mary Ann was told she would never get pregnant again. It had been devastating to her and Elmer. They had hoped God would bless them with children but He seemed to have other plans.

"It's too bad," Rachel thought. *"They would be wonderful parents."* Mary Ann could do anything. She sewed her own clothes, created the most beautiful oil paintings, could do any craft imaginable, taught piano lessons to the neighborhood children, and was a wonderful cook. Everyone loved Mary Ann and it didn't take Rachel long to share in that love.

Elmer was a quiet sort with an easy smile. It seemed as if he was always thinking about something since he listened more than he talked. Elmer and Mary Ann were so happy, always laughing and joking with each other and with Rachel.

Rachel wanted to earn her keep and had applied for more jobs than she cared to admit. The cards were stacked against her

11

because she was unmarried, pregnant, and too young to have any marketable skills. She tried her best to stay positive, but with each job that turned her down, she felt more and more rejected.

Rachel had every intention of keeping her baby. That was the plan, anyway, but reality began to close in hard around her. She was terrified. She could not even support *herself*, much less a baby. So, once again, she crouched on the floor of the closet in the corner bedroom, hugged her knees and tried to muffle her cries. Unless God worked something out quickly, she would not be able to provide for the child growing inside of her.

Mustering what little faith she still had left, Rachel cried out to God from the closet floor, told Him how much she wanted this baby and begged Him to make a way for it to happen. Night after night, month after month, she cried out to God with the same desperate plea but nothing changed. Why wasn't He answering her? Was He punishing her for stepping outside His plan and getting pregnant in the first place? *How long, O Lord? Will you forget me forever? How long will you hide your face from me? How long must I wrestle with my thoughts and every day have sorrow in my heart?* (Psalm 13:1-2, NIV).

A few days before Easter, Rachel read the scriptures leading up to crucifixion. Jesus was about to face the most painful ordeal of his life. His prayer on the Mount of Olives echoed over and over in her head. *Father, if you are willing, take this cup from me; yet not my will, but yours be done* (Luke 22:42, NIV). And then it hit her. She had been praying the wrong prayer, for *her* will to be done.

It was agonizing to even think about, much less form the words on her lips. It felt as if someone was literally grabbing her heart and pulling it out of her chest, ripping her very soul to its core.

"Lord," she managed to whisper, "I want this child more than anything in this world, but nevertheless...not *my* will but *Yours* be done."

The moment the words escaped her lips, she knew with absolute certainty that the tiny being squirming around inside of her would never be hers to keep. God had a bigger and better plan. She knew what she had to do.

A sense of relief mixed with dread washed over Rachel as she pulled up a chair next to Mary Ann, who sat gracefully behind an easel, effortlessly creating her next masterpiece with each stroke of a paintbrush. Fighting back tears, Rachel asked Mary Ann if she and Elmer would adopt the baby.

Once Rachel managed to get the words out of her mouth, she knew there was no turning back. She could never go back on her word. It would be unforgivable and unbelievably selfish to take it all back when she had given Mary Ann hope of finally becoming a mother.

Meanwhile, the Chandlers were cautious, quietly expectant. They knew Rachel could change her mind at any point. They had already lived through the pain of losing one baby and did not want to set themselves up for further heartache.

There were no obvious plans for this baby. No nursery, baby clothes or furniture. Rachel wondered if Mary Ann and Elmer really wanted this child after all or if they were sparing her a glimpse of what life would be like with the baby she had so desperately wanted but could not keep.

The baby girl was born at 12:02 a.m. on August 9th, just barely missing the due date. Rachel lifted her head long enough to see if the baby's ears were flat. Rachel's stuck out and she had always been very self conscious about it. All she saw was a head full of dark hair as nurses wrapped the baby in a blanket and whisked her out of the room. "Wait!" Rachel wanted to scream but she held back. All she could do was cry.

She never held her baby girl in her arms or even saw her face in the days that followed. Rachel had made that decision on her own, thinking it would be best if she did not have a chance to get attached to the baby. Now that it was all said and done, Rachel wondered how she could say goodbye to this little angel when she had never said hello.

A few days later, Prof Graham drove Rachel to the lawyer's office. As they pulled into the parking lot, she had a lump in her throat so big that she could not swallow, much less breathe. The only thing making this any easier was the glow on Mary Ann's face. She was so happy for Mary Ann and Elmer and did not want anything to ruin this moment for them.

Rachel felt tears well up in her eyes as she looked down at the page where she would sign her name and agree to relinquish the title of "mother" to the baby she had carried for nine months, the baby she loved more than anything. She fought back the tears and clenched her jaw so tight she thought her teeth would break, praying that God would give her the strength she needed for this moment and to please not let her fall apart in front of the Chandlers. As excruciating as it was for her, she fought hard to remain completely expressionless. She did not want to ruin this moment for them.

Rachel's signature resembled the crayon scrawling of a young child learning to write her name for the first time as she made a conscious effort not to tear the paper with the pen in her hand. Rachel stared at the page with numb disbelief as the finality of it all started to sink in. The tears she had refused to let fall now felt as if they had collected in her lungs, preventing her from drawing in breath, drowning her. At that moment she wished she *could* drown; anything to end this pain.

Loving arms wrapped themselves around Rachel and held her tight, enveloping her in the familiar scent of Mary Ann's rose scented lotion and Avon perfume.

"Thank you. This means....so much." Mary Ann whispered in Rachel's ear.

Determined to remain poised and in control, Rachel forced a smile and let herself relax in Mary Ann's arms. The Chandlers kissed Rachel goodbye and told her they loved her. Then, arm in arm, they practically floated away with smiles and laughter, papers in hand, ready to take their baby girl home. She stared after them in a daze and looked down at her own hands. Empty...just like she felt inside.

The numbness began to wear off, leaving Rachel alone with not only the physical aftermath of giving birth, but the emotional turmoil of giving up her baby. Every part of her throbbed with pain. The gallons of tears she had stuffed down deep inside began to force their way out, slowly at first like a light rain, then gradually picking up momentum as the car carried her past the city limits. She stared out the back windshield, watching the city grow smaller and smaller, leaving her baby girl, a piece of her heart, further and further behind.

"Jesus," she cried out. "Bring your comfort, Lord. Please, Father! I need to know I'm doing the right thing."

She wrapped her arms around herself and gently rocked back and forth as she sobbed. Her face was covered in a mixture of snot and tears, and her head pounded with each beat of her heart. Even so, a calming peace rushed over her as these words were clearly spoken to her spirit:

I prayed for this child and the Lord has heard me. So now I give her to the Lord. As long as she lives, she is in His safekeeping (I Samuel 1:27-28, paraphrased).

God had not answered Rachel's prayer the way she had wanted, but she knew in her heart that the baby girl she left behind was not hers, but His. The baby had been His from the moment she was conceived.

> *For you created my inmost being; you knit me together in my mother's womb. I praise you because I am fearfully and wonderfully made; your works are wonderful, I know that full well. My frame was not hidden from you when I was made in the secret place. When I was woven together in the depths of the earth, your eyes saw my unformed body. All the days ordained for me were written in your book before one of them came to be* (Psalm 139:13-16, NIV).

Mary Ann

It was well after midnight when Mary Ann slipped out of bed and quietly tiptoed down the hall. She peeked through the crack in the door at her sleeping beauty, surrounded by a watchful guard of stuffed animals, and smiled. She leaned against the doorframe and just listened to the soft, steady breathing. Mary Ann's bottom lip began to quiver and a cry almost escaped her lips, but she quickly covered her mouth with her hand. She needed a miracle. This precious child still needed her Mommy.

"I haven't loved her long enough, Lord. There are still so many things I want to experience with her. So many things I want to teach her."

Mary Ann had wanted to be a mother ever since she was a little girl. She and Elmer both loved children and wanted a houseful of them. She couldn't wait to have the deafening silence in their home drowned out by laughter and the pitter patter of little feet. The day she found out she was pregnant was the happiest day of their lives. The day her son was stillborn was one of the darkest.

Mary Ann had hosted more baby showers than she could count and though she was genuinely happy for each and every friend's blessing, there was always a hidden sadness behind her smile. She would never let anyone see it, of course, but as she packed up the punch bowl and boxed up leftover cake and mints, she would silently ask God when it would be her turn. Year after year went by with the same question and, seemingly, the same answer.

She had gone through a time of frustration, anger, depression, and even whining to God, but it didn't last long. She refused to let it. God knew she wanted a child. If it was His will for her life, He would make it happen in His own timing. If not, He was still her God, and she trusted that He knew what was best for her.

When Rachel came to stay in their home, Mary Ann knew it was by divine appointment. She and Elmer were called to love Rachel and minister to her the best they could. Mary Ann never imagined that this simple act of obedience would ultimately be the answer to years of prayer. If there had been a houseful of children like they had planned, there would not have been room to host the young, pregnant Rachel who was carrying the child God had given them to raise. Mary Ann shook her head in amazement. He is such a good God. He had not always answered her prayers the way she thought He would or in her own timeframe, but His ways were so much better.

Mary Ann kept reminding herself of this as she blew a silent kiss to her daughter and padded down the hallway into the guestroom that had taken on a new identity as a sewing nook. She carefully unfolded the thin brown tissue paper pattern and carefully pulled several pins from a tomato shaped pincushion, securing them in her teeth until they were needed.

All troubles and gloom slowly lifted as she pinned patterned shapes of a tiny dress to Strawberry Shortcake printed material and cut around the black dotted lines. It would be a size too big right now but at least her princess would have it if...just in case. She shook off the tears and converted every ounce of anxiety into focusing on her project.

There was always a project. The stillness of night left Mary Ann alone with her thoughts, leaving her in a fog of panic and fear of the unknown. Especially now. The specialist had sat her and Elmer down and told them the cancer had spread. It was inoperable. There was simply nothing more the doctors could do for her. Unless God granted her the miracle she desperately sought, Mary Ann was going to die, leaving the love of her life to raise their little girl alone. The thought was more than Mary Ann could bear, so she busied herself with projects – sewing, painting, ceramics, cooking - anything to put her mind at ease.

The last project had come late in the summer. Mary Ann and Elmer always had a garden in their oversized backyard. It was something they both enjoyed, watching the tiny seeds they had planted turn into a bountiful harvest. That particular summer the garden produced an abundance of green beans and it had taken hours to pick them. She and Elmer had collapsed at the dining room table afterward, covered in soil and stared at the crates full of beans, wondering aloud what they would do with it all.

Elmer awoke in the middle of the night and noticed Mary Ann wasn't in bed. Concerned that she wasn't feeling well, he got up and found her standing over a hot stove with canning jars.

"Honey, what are you *doing*?" he had asked, staring in amazement at the countertop overflowing with glass jars of green beans. "This is more than we'll ever be able to eat."

Without missing a beat, she said, "I want my baby girl to have fresh green beans and I don't know how much longer I will feel up to doing this."

Silly? Maybe, but at least Mary Ann knew her daughter would have special, handmade clothes and good food. She would be taken care of – at least for a while.

After cutting the last half-circle for the Strawberry Shortcake dress, Mary Ann took a deep breath, closed her eyes and turned her face toward the ceiling.

"I know you will take care of her, Father. After all, she's not mine. She's yours."

It was as if she had opened a window of her soul, letting a fresh breeze of peace wash over her. God had heard her. She remembered the scripture engraved on the plaque that hung under her little girl's portrait in the entryway, a portrait Mary Ann had painted before the cancer. She could not think of words more perfect to express her heart at that moment: *I prayed for this child, and the Lord has granted me what I asked of him. So now I give [her] to the Lord. For [her] whole life [she] will be given over to the Lord* (I Samuel 1:27-28, NIV).

Mary Ann had wanted this precious child so much for so long that it was hard to fathom handing her over to someone else's care. Yet Mary Ann knew without a shadow of a doubt that no one loved her baby girl more than Jesus, and she would be safe in His arms.

"Take care of my baby," she whispered aloud.

Years of Bible study and scripture memorization had brought her so much comfort in the times of her deepest need. She opened the small, tattered red Bible to the Book of Psalms where she had recently highlighted this passage:

Give ear to my words, O Lord, consider my sighing. Listen to my cry for help, my king and my God, for to you I pray. In the morning, O Lord, you hear my voice; in the morning I lay my requests before you and wait in expectation (Psalm 5:1-3, NIV).

She closed her eyes and silently thanked God for His word, which always offered the exact encouragement she needed. Then, swallowing the lump that had formed in her throat, Mary Ann gathered up the pieces of the Strawberry Shortcake dress. She threaded the bobbin of her sewing machine and carefully guided the material, letting the whir of the needle drown out any residual sadness as she began what would be her final sewing project, and quietly sang her favorite hymn in praise and adoration.

"When Christ shall come, with shout of acclamation
And take me home, what joy shall fill my heart!
Then I shall bow in humble adoration
And there proclaim, 'My God, how great Thou art!'
Then sings my soul, my Savior God to Thee
How great Thou art! How great Thou art!" [1]

---

[1] Hines, Stuart. *How Great Thou Art.* Manna Music, 1953. Public domain.

Clair Chandler Rivera

My Three Moms

It's lunch hour on a Friday and I'm holding up the line at my local bank. All I want to do is make a quick withdrawal so I can run to Schlotzsky's® and pick up the sandwich I had strategically called in fifteen minutes ago - the sandwich I had been looking forward to all day. It was probably soggy and cold by now. In my haste to leave the office I forgot my ID and was now forced to ramble off account numbers, social security number, drivers license number, all of which had been dedicated to memory years ago. It was the next question that had me stumped.

"And your mother's maiden name?"

My mind went blank. Which name had I given them *this* time? Rachel's? Mary Ann's? Or was it my stepmother, Darlene's? I considered each of them to be my mother and had grown to loathe that particular security question.

"*You need to just pick one and stick with it,*" I sternly thought to myself.

The lady behind me began to sigh loudly. "For the love..." she muttered under her breath.

I leaned forward with both hands on the counter and whispered the three choices as I almost apologetically explained that I have three moms. The teller raised one eyebrow, but my answer must have satisfied her. Cash in hand, I ducked my head and made a quick departure, hiding behind the bank envelope that I strategically held at my temple in order to avoid eye contact with the other patrons. *Note to self: use the drive-thru from now on.*

22

I have never been sure how to handle the "mom dilemma." It is so confusing, even to me, that I often wish I had a pocket-sized flow chart and a laser pointer to explain the chain of events that had made me a daughter to not just one but three different women.

I rarely thought about my birthmother growing up, although, admittedly a small part of my life was often a question mark. I had always known I was adopted, or at least I cannot remember *not* knowing. It was never a real issue. Rachel gave birth to me and I respected her for that, but it takes so much more to be a parent. My *parents* were the ones who got up with me in the middle of the night when I was sick. They were the ones sitting on the front row for every piano recital and school play. They held me when I was sad or hurt. They made sacrifices so that I could go to camp and later on, college. *They* were responsible for the person I had become. Not *her*.

Nevertheless, I sometimes wondered if I looked like Rachel or laughed like her. I sometimes longed just to see her, if only from a distance. I wondered where I came from and quite possibly, what I was spared from. Once in a while, in the stillness of night when I was somewhere between sleep and awake, I would wonder what she was doing now: if she had other children, if she was happy, if she thought about me on my birthday...or if she thought of me at *all*.

As for Mary Ann, I really wish I remembered more about her but my memories are jumbled with random blips, like an old, spliced home movie on a projector screen. I was six years old when I remember hearing the name to her strange illness. The chemotherapy left her weak and frail. The most vivid memories I have of her involve IV needles, vomiting, wigs, and hospital rooms. I feel guilty about it now, but I would beg my dad not to make me visit her anymore. I felt helpless, scared and even nauseated to see the once vibrant young woman resemble a Halloween skeleton with a thin, bruised layer of skin tightly stretched over it. When she held my hand, I could see every vein, every tendon.

I remember the night my dad sat me down to tell me the cancer had progressed and unless God decided to work a miracle, Mommy was going to heaven to be with Jesus. I had never seen my dad cry until that night. I sat in his lap, holding a stuffed lamb he had given me just before our talk. It had a wind up music box inside of it that played "Brahms's Lullaby" when I turned the silver key on the side. I clung to that lamb as if it were a life preserver in this overwhelming sea of grief that I had been so abruptly dumped into.

"No!" I screamed over and over again. "Jesus will fix her! He *will!*"

I began to kick, scream, and cry. I tore myself away from my dad and curled up on a nearby couch, turning my back toward him. Why would he say such an awful thing? More importantly, why wasn't Jesus doing anything for Mommy? I knew He could if He wanted to. I didn't understand, so I kept holding on to the stuffed lamb as I tried to hold on to my faith, winding it up again when the music began to fade.

It wasn't long after that night when Mary Ann lost the battle to the cancerous poison in her body. I knew it was coming, but that didn't stop the numbing, debilitating feeling of knowing I would never see her again on this earth.

I was told that she was better off with Jesus and I wanted to believe that. Part of me was secretly relieved that Mommy was finally free from pain. I pictured her running barefoot through grassy meadows in heaven. She had her own hair, not a synthetic mass of curls. Her face was rosy instead of yellow, her eyes bright sunbeams instead of dull pools. She was a healthy weight, even a little bit on the plump side. She was running, laughing and picking flowers.

The other part of me was still angry with God. How could I trust Him to take good care of my mom when I could no longer trust in His promises or His ability to heal?

Life had to go on without her. It seemed almost crass. The world should have stopped spinning the very moment Mary Ann departed from it. Wall Street should have shut down. The sun should have refused to shine. President Reagan should have declared a National Day of Mourning. Instead, children played in the park. Couples walked arm in arm. People packed into restaurants, talking and laughing. How dare they? Didn't they know the most important woman in my world had died?

A year later, my dad started dating Darlene, a woman he met at church. Petite and strikingly beautiful with perfectly coifed hair, I liked her right away. It was hard at first to see my dad with someone other than my mom. At the same time, a burden lifted from my shoulders since I no longer felt solely responsible for his happiness.

I was afraid to allow another woman into my life, but as much as I hated to admit it, I desperately needed a mother. No one could ever take Mary Ann's place, but I knew that even Mary

Ann would want me to have the guidance and nurturing that only a woman could give.

So in a pink and white striped dress, I sat in the front row of the church I had grown up in and watched my dad pledge his love and affection to the woman who would move into our home and become my new mom. Mom number three. I couldn't wait for them to get back from their honeymoon so I could be like all the other girls in my third grade class who had moms - staying up late on Friday nights doing things like painting our toenails or piling under blankets on the living room floor, watching movies and eating popcorn. I wanted someone to teach me how to be a lady, to show me how to fix my hair and put on makeup and teach me about fashion; someone who would be there after school to sit at the kitchen table and give me her undivided attention as I told her every detail of my day over a glass of milk; someone I could tell my secrets to.

Though she did the best she could under the circumstances, the reality of the situation was that Darlene already had a lot of other people, mostly elderly family members, depending on her for their care. More often than not, I came home to an empty house to find a note on the table as to her whereabouts.

So while other little girls my age expressed hopes and dreams of growing up to become a mom, that was the *last* thing I wanted to be. In the first six years of my life, two mothers had already checked out on me: Rachel, for reasons I did not understand at the time; Mary Ann, because God was mean, or at least that was the case in my young mind; and now, it seemed Darlene was too busy for me. I decided to pass on the idea of becoming a mother the way one might pass the Brussels sprouts at the dinner table. Motherhood might satisfy someone else's hungering desire, but so far it had only left a bad taste in my mouth.

My Own Journey

Ten years later, I had not changed my mind. I came to college with many hopes and dreams, but none of them included being a mom. I wanted to travel, have an exciting career and live spontaneously...at least that's what I *thought* I wanted.

By my junior year in college, most of my friends were either engaged or already married. Suddenly the thought of being alone was utterly terrifying. I was stricken with fear that if something didn't happen soon, I would be alone for the rest of my life, knitting in a recliner and surrounded by a houseful of cats.

Nathan* and I had known each other since junior high, and he had recently transferred to the college I attended. I thought he was sweet and a far better person than I could ever hope to be. He was everything I thought I "should" want in a man and I knew he was crazy about me.

It was a whirlwind romance, if you want to call it that, and Nathan and I were engaged two months after we started dating. Everyone thought we were a perfect match. Nathan and I had grown up together. We knew the same people and had attended the same schools. Most importantly to me at the time, my family loved Nathan, something that carried a lot more weight than I probably should have let it.

The problem was that *I* did not love Nathan. At least not the way a wife should love her husband. The truth was that the marriage was already troubled before it ever started, riddled with lies and ulterior motives, founded on a sense of obligation rather than mutual attraction, respect and love. One month before the wedding, I knew I should call the whole thing off and walk – no, *run* – away but I was young, insecure, and continually striving to achieve the unattainable goal of making everyone else happy.

So on a cold December afternoon, I walked down the aisle of a packed church, pale and much too thin. Three layers of blush caked my cheeks, sunken and sallow from months of dealing with a nervous stomach. Thick concealer attempted to erase the dark circles under my eyes from lack of sleep. The designer dress that had once fit like a glove gaped around my arms, waist, and bust line. With each step closer to Nathan, I told myself that everyone got cold feet on their wedding day, and that there were no perfect marriages. It was going to be O.K. It *had* to be.

I think we had been married for a whole five minutes when people began asking us when we were going to have a baby. Nathan and I had discussed it prior to the engagement and there would be no baby. Not now. Not ever. As you can probably imagine, that didn't exactly go over well with a lot of people. Our reproductive decisions suddenly became everyone else's business:

"You don't *ever* want to have a baby?"

"Oh, you'll change your mind."

"Do you not *like* babies?"

"Doesn't Nathan want to have his name carried down?"

"How sad for your parents."

Our decision not to have children was sometimes considered selfish and even "liberal" in one church we attended, whose name and denomination will remain anonymous. I'm still not entirely sure how we ended up in this particular Sunday school class or why we stayed. I have never felt so out of place in my life than I did in what I affectionately referred to as the

"Biblical Twilight Zone." It was chock-full of stay-at-home moms who would refer to me in hushed tones as "the one who works," as if saying "the one with contagious dysentery. Don't get too close or it may rub off on you."

I was an outsider, unable to participate in Mothers of Preschoolers meetings on Tuesday mornings or possessing any sort of desire to work a childcare shift in the nursery. While others would *ooh* and *aah* over the new babies that seemed to appear at least once every quarter to couples in our age group, my general opinion was that 'you've seen one baby, you've seen them all.' I did not want to hold new babies, go to anyone else's baby shower, listen to the gory details of anyone's labor and delivery, or learn about hospital grade breast pumps. I wanted to discuss things that truly mattered in my world – tax reform, ways to improve the criminal justice system, equal pay for equal work, social programs to empower the underprivileged...but when I raised such topics, the other women looked at me like I was speaking Urdu.

While I felt like a complete outcast around these women, I began to wonder if they were on to something. They all appeared to have happy marriages, which was something I desperately wanted but lacked.

By this time, Nathan and I had been married for six years, but barely hanging on for the last four. We were little more than great roommates. We enjoyed each other's company for the most part and rarely had conflict, but not because there was nothing to fight about. So *much* was wrong that we didn't know where to start. Maybe having a baby was exactly what we needed to get our relationship back on track. It was at least worth a shot.

Nathan reluctantly agreed, though he thought a baby would only make things "more complicated."

We tried to get pregnant for six months, something else I had not expected. I thought that once we decided to have a baby, I would just get off the pill and it would happen right away. At least that is how it seemed to work for everyone around me.

"Your body is not like everyone else's," my doctor had tried to explain when I expressed my frustrations. "It may not happen for you. Endometriosis is not exactly conducive to pregnancy."

Still, I was determined. I knew other people with endometriosis who had gotten pregnant and I earnestly believed this was God's will, both for me and my marriage.

Month after month, I rushed to the drug store for an early pregnancy test, too impatient to wait until I was actually "late." I kept myself busy by reorganizing the medicine cabinets for the two minutes, which felt more like two *hours*, it took to get a result. Even when the test was clearly negative, I refused to believe it. I held on to hope until the moment I started my period and then fell apart, crumbling in a heap and sobbing alone on the bathroom floor.

And then the day came. It was mid-November, 2002, and time to take another test. I imagined what it would be like to announce I was pregnant over Thanksgiving dinner. Nathan's family had a tradition where each person at the table shared what they were thankful for. Wouldn't that be the perfect opportunity to share the news? I imagined the squeals of delight followed by laughter and hugs as the family patted my belly and slapped Nathan on the back. *Sigh.*

31

I glanced over at the test and winced, fully expecting to see one bright pink line staring back at me. But wait? What's this? Is that a second pink line? The line was faint, but it was definitely there.

"Guess what?" I shrieked, bursting through the bathroom door with the test in my hand.

"You're pregnant," Nathan said flatly. "Congratulations."

There was barely a hint of excitement in his voice and the ear-to-ear grin that had adorned my face slowly began to fade like a deflating balloon.

"Yeah. Uh, thanks."

I bit my bottom lip and spun around on my heel so Nathan wouldn't see the single tear making its way down my cheek. I quickly wiped it away with the back of my hand and told myself he was as happy as I was, but deep inside I knew better.

Everyone thought we were the perfect couple with a fairytale marriage. Everyone, that is, but my friend, Jennifer. I was so relieved when Jennifer and her husband, Brian, joined our church because I finally had an ally in enemy territory, a.k.a. the Biblical Twilight Zone Sunday school class. Jennifer also worked outside the home (*gasp, horror*).

Someone once said that a person is lucky to have three close, genuine friends in a lifetime. Up to that point in my life, I only had one: Kelly, my best friend from high school. I had many acquaintances and was actually quite social, but I held most people at arm's length and made a point not to let anyone in. I had been hurt one too many times to let myself be that vulnerable again. Jennifer soon broke through the barrier around my heart and I considered her my second true friend.

So while everyone else may have crowned me and Nathan "couple of the year," Jennifer didn't buy it for a minute, even *before* she knew all of our dirty laundry. She thought we looked more like a pair of badly mismatched socks.

"I never in a million years would have put you two together. You remind me of Doug and Carrie from *The King of Queens*," she once said matter-of-factly, "only *they* kind of work. You and Nathan don't at all."

Jennifer knew my marriage was barely hanging by a thread and the only reason I wanted this baby so badly is because it would be the one thing that would convince me to stay. I called her as soon as I got to work to tell her the news, knowing I would get the response I was looking for. I was right. Jennifer, who had recently learned she was pregnant as well, was beside herself with excitement.

We normally talked at least three or four times a day anyway, but now our conversations took on new meaning. Our babies would be best friends just like us. We had another excuse to spend more time together. When Nathan grew even more distant with the news of my pregnancy, Jennifer stepped up to support me. I honestly did not know what I would have done without her.

Then the unthinkable happened. I noticed some tiny drops of blood and panicked. I called my doctor, who assured me that a little bit of bleeding was normal and as long as I had no cramping or clotting everything was probably fine. It had not occurred to me that anything could possibly go wrong. I thought once I was pregnant I would stay that way for the full nine months and then hold a precious baby in my arms. I was not at all prepared for what was to come.

Two days later, the Sunday morning before Thanksgiving, I woke up in so much pain that I was doubled over and moaning. The tiny droplets had turned into bright red clots. Terrified, I called my doctor again, who told me to keep my feet elevated and come in the following morning for an exam; however, there was nothing that could be done this early in the pregnancy to prevent me from losing the baby.

The next call I made was to Jennifer. All I could say was, "I'm bleeding and I'm scared" before bursting into tears. There was a long silence on the other end of the line and then my sweet friend did the only thing she knew to do. She began to pray.

"Lord Jesus, we come to you right now and ask you to bring healing. We know you love this baby and we ask for your protection over this pregnancy and over Clair right now. We love you and we trust you."

As Jennifer prayed, I pleaded with God to hear her and to hear my heart. I asked Him to forgive the inner vows I had made as a young child that I never wanted to be a mother. *I didn't mean it, Lord. I didn't know...*

But the bleeding did not slow down. It got worse. A sonogram the following morning confirmed my fears. An empty womb. An empty heart. Empty to the point of numbness.

My mind was a dense fog for weeks afterward. Life went on all around me and I was angry about that. I was angry at the casual "it happens" attitude of the doctor. I was angry at Nathan, who had casually shrugged and only said, "Hey, I'm sorry," after the nurse had left us alone with our thoughts following the sonogram. I was angry that the loss of my child was reduced to a checkmark on a medical form as a "spontaneous abortion." I was angry at the happy pregnant women with swollen bellies that I passed in the lobby on the way out of the doctor's office, smiling and sharing sonogram pictures. I wanted to scream at them. How could anyone possibly smile when my unborn child would never have that opportunity?

My cell phone rang as we walked to the elevators outside the lobby, bringing me back to reality. I glanced down at the caller ID and saw that it was Jennifer. *Oh, God.* I lost all control of my emotions as I stared at the phone. I knew everything was about to change in my friendship with Jennifer. I thrust the phone at Nathan, sobbing and shaking my head. I couldn't talk to her. He took several steps away from me and talked in hushed tones. With his hand over the receiver, he asked if I wanted her to come over. I shook my head "no" and sobbed even louder. Jennifer was the *last* person I wanted to see at that moment. The thought of having her hug me with a tiny bump in between us was more than I could handle.

I no longer knew how to relate to Jennifer. I was so used to sharing everything with her but now things were so different. I felt like I couldn't possibly share the depth of my anguish and bitterness. This was a time in her life to be celebrating and I didn't feel like celebrating. I couldn't even *pretend* to be happy for her. I refused her phone calls and offers to come over and comfort me. Slowly but surely, I withdrew not only from Jennifer but from Nathan, my family and ultimately, God. I was reduced to a shell of a person, wallowing in misery and self-pity.

Chapter 2: Hannah's Prayer

In the midst of everything I had been going through, I did what most of us do when we're mad at God. I quit spending time in His word and stopped talking to Him altogether unless it was to complain or yell at Him. I folded my arms, furrowed my brow and pouted like a spoiled four-year-old child instead of running with open arms to the only One who could bring me comfort and peace in the midst of my circumstances. The irony was that I had only punished myself by pushing God away. I could hear the voice of Dr. Phil asking, "And how's that workin' for ya?" It wasn't. It never does.

When I began to open my Bible again, I found numerous counts of women who were unable to have a child for one reason or another. Many of them come straight out of Genesis and may be familiar to you:

- Sarah – *The Lord has kept me from having children* (Genesis 16:2, NIV);
- Rebekah – *Isaac prayed to the Lord on behalf of his wife, because she was barren* (Genesis 25:21, NIV);
- Leah – *When the Lord saw that Leah was not loved, he opened her womb* (Genesis 29:31, NIV);
- Rachel – *Then God remembered Rachel; he listened to her and opened her womb* (Genesis 30:22, NIV).

A little deeper into the Old Testament is where I connected with a kindred spirit, someone I totally related to. I think you'll like her, too. Her story encouraged me, gave me hope, and inspired me to keep trusting God for a baby. Her name is Hannah. Of all the women mentioned in the Bible who struggled with fertility issues, Hannah is the only one who gives us a glimpse into the longings of her heart. I spent hours with her as I poured through the first chapter of I Samuel:

There was a man named Elkanah...[who] had two wives, Hannah and Peninnah. Peninnah had children, but Hannah did not (I Samuel 1:1-2).

The chapter starts out by introducing Hannah's husband, Elkanah, and the fact that he had two wives, something that was very common in those days, Penninah and Hannah. Penninah had children (notice the plural), but Hannah had none.

Let's put that in today's context. Fortunately we no longer live in a society where polygamy is the norm. However, if you are in the same difficult season in your life as Hannah was, it may seem like every woman in your life is blessed with a child – sometimes a whole gaggle of them – and it makes you feel ten times worse.

> *So Peninnah would taunt Hannah and make fun of her because the Lord had kept her from having children. Year after year it was the same – Peninnah would taunt Hannah as they went to the Tabernacle. Each time, Hannah would be reduced to tears and would not even eat*
> (I Samuel 1:6-7).

Put yourself in Hannah's shoes for a minute. Think about something you are very self conscious about that you cannot change. Maybe it's the size of your nose, a scar, an injury, a deformity, or even something about your family background. Now imagine how you would feel if your biggest competitor used it to torment you.

Hannah already felt like less than a woman because she was barren. It was one thing for *her* to feel that way. It was quite another to have it constantly rubbed in her face by "the other woman." Penninah wasn't just a woman that Hannah saw only once or twice a week at church, or even someone she had to spend eight hours a day with at work. Penninah shared both Hannah's home and her husband. There was no running away from her. Day in and day out, Hannah was face to face with Penninah, a woman who had the children Hannah longed for. Doesn't your heart just break for Hannah? I know mine does.

What makes it even worse is that Penninah *knew* how badly Hannah wanted children but rather than making a concerted effort to treat the matter with sensitivity, she rubbed Hannah's face in it year after year (v.7). Every waking hour of every day, year after year, Hannah was not only reminded of the empty crib in the nursery, but *taunted* about it by the woman with whom she had to share both her home and her husband. I can think of no greater pain. It makes me wonder what kind of insecurities and hurts Penninah must have carried to cause her to be so mean to Hannah. As a matter of fact, the New International Version® of the Bible doesn't even call Penninah by name after verse four. She is referred to only as Hannah's "rival" (v. 6, 7).

I sincerely hope you have not been the victim of a Penninah in your own struggle with having a child. People can say and do the meanest things sometimes, though most of it is unintentional.

A woman in my Sunday school class, a mother of two beautiful children, called me shortly after my first miscarriage in an attempt to offer her condolences. I was horrified when she very matter-of-factly stated that "some people just aren't meant to be parents." As terrible as it was, I honestly don't think she meant her thoughtless comment to be hurtful.

Penninah, on the other hand, said cruel things like this to Hannah with full knowledge that her words would absolutely crush Hannah's heart. Scripture says Penninah continually pushed Hannah's buttons and emotionally tortured her until Hannah "wept and would not eat" (v.7).

I think there is a big difference between crying and weeping. The fact that Hannah *wept* indicates more than bloodshot eyes and a few tears streaking her cheeks. She was *broken* – the deepest, innermost part of her soul deeply wounded. I picture Hannah curled up on her bed, sobbing uncontrollably until her chest ached and her head began to throb. The *ugly* cry. I can relate to that.

To make matters worse, Hannah's husband, the person closest to her, tries to minimize what she's going through: *"Why are you crying, Hannah?" Elkanah would ask. "Why aren't you eating? Why be downhearted just because you have no children? You have me – isn't that better than having ten sons?"* (I Samuel 1:8).

I'm sure Elkanah meant well. Scripture indicates that he loved Hannah (v. 5). I think the poor guy just didn't know *what* to say and either had one of those moments where it sounded better in his head than it did out loud, or opened his mouth to say something comforting and that's just what came out. Either way, the next verse does not indicate that Hannah was comforted by his words or suddenly snapped out of the funk she was in. In all likelihood, she probably felt worse than she did before.

When word got out that I had miscarried, the people in my life really wanted to offer me comfort and hope. I sincerely believe that. What came out of their *mouths*, however, was not a true reflection of what was in their hearts, and ended up being very hurtful. This is just a sample of the things that were said (and great examples of what *not* to say to someone who has gone through a miscarriage):

"There was probably something wrong with the baby."

"Just try again in three months."

"I heard that caffeine causes miscarriage, so it was probably that cup of coffee."

"The baby probably sensed that you were stressed and didn't want to add to that."

"One in four pregnancies ends in miscarriage."

"At least it was in the early stages and didn't look like a real baby yet."

"It's been a whole week already, so why aren't you over it yet?"

Or the absolute *worst* thing that was ever said to me that I mentioned earlier:

"Some people just aren't meant to be parents".

My Sunday school teacher actually had the nerve to suggest that if I would have allowed him to lay hands on me and pray over me when I was pregnant this never would have happened. *What miserable comforters you are!* (Job 16:2).

Here's a free piece of advice: when you don't have the right words to say to someone who is hurting, do not try to cheer them up or say you understand when you really don't have a clue. Do not try to compare losses or get overly spiritual. Simply say, "I love you. I'm sorry you're hurting. Please let me know if there is something I can do to make this easier for you."

Hannah had no one to sympathize with her. No one seemed to understand what she was going through or cared enough about her to find out. She was in a far worse position that I had ever been. *Hannah was in deep anguish, crying bitterly as she prayed to the Lord. And she made this vow: "O Lord of Heaven's Armies, if you will look upon my sorrow and answer my prayer and give me a son, then I will give him back to you* (I Samuel 1:10-11).

In deep anguish and crying bitterly. Hannah was in a very dark place that many of us can probably relate to. No happiness or joy could be found anywhere within the depths of her soul. She had a constant ringing in her ears and a steady pounding in her head from hours upon hours of crying. Every ounce of energy she could muster was quickly zapped by pure exhaustion. Everything around her, no matter how vibrant and colorful, looked dingy gray. Every morsel she put in her mouth, no matter how rich or delicious, was bland, tasteless, or bitter. The fragrances around her, no matter how sweet, smelled faintly of stench.

Like Hannah, most women want to be mothers at some point in their life. Part of what makes us uniquely female is the ability to nurture new life from the womb and beyond. The inability to have a baby, whether through infertility or miscarriage, can be devastating. It goes against our very design.

In talking to other women who have struggled in this area, a lot of different words were used to describe how it made them feel: defective, inadequate, disappointed, frustrated, incomplete, forgotten, and desperate. If you do not know who you are in Christ, these lies can quickly take root. Like weeds, they will take over your thoughts and choke out the truth of God's word, sending you to a place of spiritual emptiness where you do not want to be (more on that in the next section). The greatest "weed killer" you have is *the sword of the Spirit, which is the word of God* (Ephesians 6:17).

Start by replacing any thoughts that make you feel like anything other than a daughter of the King until you can say with bold confidence:

I am *not* defective. I am *fearfully* and *wonderfully* made (Psalm 139:14, emphasis added).

I am *not* inadequate. I can do *everything* through Him who gives me strength (Philippians 4:13, emphasis added).

I may *feel* disappointed, but I have *hope* through Jesus Christ and this hope *does not* disappoint (Romans 5:5, emphasis added).

I don't *have* to be frustrated because what is impossible with men *is possible* with God (Luke 18:27, emphasis added).

I am *not* incomplete. God has blessed me with *every spiritual blessing in the heavenly realms* because I am united with Christ; therefore I have everything I need to live in victory (Ephesians 1:3, emphasis added).

I am *not* forgotten. God has written *my name* on the palms of His hand (Isaiah 49:16, emphasis added).

I will *no longer* feel desperate. Instead, I will give all my worries
and cares to God because *He cares about me*
(I Peter 5:7, emphasis added).

*[L]et God transform you into a new person by changing the
way you think. Then you will learn to know God's will for you,
which is good and pleasing and perfect* (Romans 12:2).

*[L]et the Spirit renew your thoughts and attitudes. Put on your
new nature, created to be like God – truly righteous and holy*
(Ephesians 4:23).

*Fix your thoughts on what is true, and honorable, and right,
and pure, and lovely, and admirable. Think about things that
are excellent and worthy of praise* (Philippians 4:8).

Part II: The Pit of Despair

*I waited patiently for the Lord to help me,
and he turned to me and heard my cry.
He lifted me out of the pit of despair,
out of the mud and the mire.
He set my feet on solid ground and
steadied me as I walked along*
(Psalm 40:1-2, emphasis added).

Either the well was very deep or she fell very slowly.
"Alice in Wonderland," Lewis Carroll

Chapter 3: Tales from the Pit

What do you think of when you hear the word 'pit'? Some of the definitions I came across sent chills down my spine: *a sizeable hole, usually in the ground; hell: the abode of Satan's forces of evil; a trap in the form of a concealed hole.*[2]

The house I grew up in had a storm cellar in the backyard. It was hidden away, concealed in ivy and wild vines. The lid was heavy, hard to open, and made a creaky sound when opened. A damp, musty smell of mildew wafted up from the deep, dark hole beneath the earth's surface. Sixteen thin metal steps with bits of rust on the edges led down into a shadowy chasm. A thick metal circular opening, like a carnival "fun house," greeted visitors on the left.

A single light bulb hung from the short ceiling and swayed ever so slightly; though from what type of air circulation is still unclear to me. Two twin-sized beds hung by chains on each wall with a bench seat positioned in between. Shelving units housed a battery operated radio and my mother's canned fruits and vegetables so we wouldn't starve to death in case we were ever in there longer than we planned.

Fortunately, I only remember going into the cellar once or twice. It was scary down there. To a little girl with a wild imagination, it was an abysmal tomb; the dwelling place of trolls, monsters and creepy critters with fangs and an appetite for human flesh. I had nightmares of being down there alone, trying to claw my way out because someone had closed the lid and put a heavy weight on top of it.

---

[2] http://www.thefreedictionary.com/pit

Another great depiction of a pit is seen in the movie, *The Princess Bride.* The hero, Westley, wakes up in a dark, strange place and is chained to a table. A ghastly character, known only as "The Albino," stands over Westley and quietly cleans his wounds.

Westley: "Where am I?"

The Albino: (raspy, sinister voice) "The pit of despair. Don't even think about (clears throat, voice changes)... don't even think about trying to escape. The chains are far too thick. And don't dream about getting rescued either. The only way in is secret. Only the Prince, the Count and I know how to get in and out."

Westley: "Then I'm here until I die?"

The Albino: "Until they kill you, yeah."[3]

Call me crazy, but there are some pretty sound theological parallels in this scene. It may take a stretch of the imagination to see them, but they may become clearer in light of the Biblical account of the demon-possessed man:

> "When Jesus stepped ashore, he was met by a demon-possessed man from the town. For a long time this man had not worn clothes or lived in a house, but had lived in the tombs. When he saw Jesus, he cried out and fell at his feet, shouting at the top of his voice, "What do you want with me, Jesus, Son of the Most High God? I beg you, don't torture me!" For Jesus had commanded the evil spirit to come out of the man. Many times it had seized him, and though he was *chained hand and foot* and *kept under guard*, he had broken his

---

[3] Reiner, Rob. <u>The Princess Bride</u>. MGM Studios, 1987.

46

chains and had been driven by the demon into *solitary places*" (Luke 8:27-29, NIV, emphasis added).

Together, these stories paint a picture of what it means to not only be in a *physical* pit, but a *spiritual* one. Using the emphasized phrases in the above scripture, we can discern some of the characteristics of a spiritual pit. Both Westley and the demon possessed man were immobilized by three key factors.

1. *Chained hand and foot*. The chains may not be visible to the naked eye, but they are there. Thick, cold metal chains with locks act as a spiritual straitjacket like the one worn by Marley in *A Christmas Carol*[4]. A heaviness of both heart and spirit are constant weights that cannot be shaken free. Others may have told you to simply "snap out of it" or "get over it" and you *want* to; but, like Westley, the chains are too thick and you are bound too tightly.

2. *Kept under guard*. A dark rain cloud follows you around all day, every day – like the dirt cloud that follows "Pig Pen" in the *Peanuts*™ cartoon. For a brief moment it may seem as if the sun is about to break through the cloud, but the moment quickly fades. You feel alone except for the cold presence of one who is out to destroy you. Like "The Albino" in the scene from *The Princess Bride*, the enemy may temporarily soothe your wounded heart with lies in order to gain your trust long enough to deceive and betray you.

3. *Driven to solitary places*. You not only feel alone in your hurt, but you have isolated yourself from the people in your life. You feel a strange sense of security within the walls of your

---

[4] Dickens, Charles. <u>A Christmas Carol</u>. Chicago: Rand McNally, 1912.

home and prefer to retreat there...alone. You refuse to accept phone calls or lunch invitations. If you're like I was, you spend much of your free time crying in bed or moping on the couch in front of the TV. Even if you are in a crowd of people, you feel totally and completely alone.

The Bible contains other stories of fellow pit dwellers, including some names you may recognize. Take Jonah, for example. In an attempt to run away from God, Jonah found himself aboard a ship in the midst of a violent storm that threatened to take the lives of everyone aboard (Jonah 1:1-5). The chains of Jonah's disobedience weighed him down as he realized he could never run from the watchful eye of God. Jonah volunteered to be thrown overboard, hoping to spare the lives of his shipmates, only to be swallowed by a huge fish (Jonah 1:12, 15-17). Jonah spent three days and three nights – 72 hours – in solitary confinement...inside the stomach of a fish (Jonah 1:12, 15 -17). Talk about muck and mire. I don't know about you, but I am so thankful God chose Jonah for this object lesson in obedience and not me! That must have been one nasty pit: dark, smelly, stuck in who-knows-what with no way out.

And then there was Joseph with his "coat of many colors" whose pride ultimately led to his downfall. Already hated for being the favorite son, Joseph made the mistake of telling his older brothers about his dreams – dreams that they were bowing down before him (Genesis 37:3-12). His cockiness only landed him in a pit. Joseph was thrown into a deep, empty well in the middle of the desert by his brothers (Genesis 37:17-24). With no ladder and no way to grip the walls of the cistern to climb out, all

Joseph could do was peer up at the hint of light coming from the opening and pray that someone would hear his cries for help.

Frustrated, exhausted, and running out of hope, he eventually stopped fighting and silently accepted his fate. "So this is how I die," Joseph thought to himself. Somewhere deep inside, a still, small voice encouraged him to hold on to hope and fight back...but he was too emotionally and physically spent to even lift his head, much less his hands.

In the weeks that followed my first miscarriage, I found myself in a pit much more terrifying than the backyard cellar could ever be. The darkness was overwhelming: nothing but thick, black, metal walls everywhere I turned. I did not climb into it voluntarily; yet, strangely, I have no recollection of being pushed into it against my will. If I had any sense of awareness about what was happening to me, I might have fought harder to keep my head above ground. Instead, I hit the bottom with a harsh thud and couldn't even pretend to know where I was or how to get out.

My slow descent into the pit began with isolation. I grew more and more reclusive because everywhere I went there were pregnant women and babies – lots of them. They seemed to strategically place themselves at the grocery store, post office, bank, church, and every restaurant I walked into. They were everywhere; following me, taunting me, and tearing my heart out.

Suddenly it seemed as if everyone Nathan and I knew was either pregnant or had recently given birth. Friends that we had not heard from in years were crawling out of the woodwork, leaving messages on our answering machine or sending birth announcements telling of the latest addition to their families. I counted six new babies in the month of December and I received four baby shower invitations in one week.

Even Christmas, my favorite time of year, was all about a baby. I didn't want Nathan to even put our tree up. I covered my ears when I heard "Away in a Manger." Everywhere I turned I felt as if I were being slapped in the face with babies, babies and more babies.

I was angry, bitter, and spiraling into a frightening state of depression. I was so consumed with grief and despair that I literally thought I was going to die. I spent days in bed with the curtains drawn, not eating or showering, doing little more than feeling sorry for myself and crying out, "Why?" As a probation officer, I saw so many people who weren't fit to be parents reproducing like rabbits yet God couldn't give me *one* child? What was *wrong* with Him? What was wrong with *me*?

I fell for the lies the enemy continually whispered in my mind: *'You will never have a baby of your own. It will always happen for everyone else in your life, but never for you. You will never feel better than you do right now. You will never be whole. God has forgotten you. Your faith has gotten you nowhere. God has turned His back on you so why don't you turn your back on Him?'* I believed every word. I allowed myself to lose all hope, all confidence in God.

How God Uses the Pit

The thing about hitting rock bottom is that there is nowhere to look but up. Joseph's experience in the pit turned his pride into humility. He no longer boasted about himself but of the Lord (Genesis 40:8, 41:16). The entire chain of events, including the pit and slavery, became part of a divine plan to place Joseph in a place of leadership within the Egyptian palace (Genesis 39-40). There, he would rise to royal position and save literally thousands of lives, including those of the brothers who had once left him for dead (Genesis 41-45).

Jonah's disobedience landed him in the pit of a whale. If God wanted to get Jonah's attention, mission accomplished. Jonah matured more in his faith in those three days than he had in his everyday life as a prophet. It took the pit to turn Jonah's heart back to the Lord. He prayed this prayer *while he was still inside the fish*: "In my distress I called to the Lord, and he answered me. From the depths of the grave I called for help, and you listened to my cry...you brought my life up from the pit, O Lord my God" (Jonah 2:2, 6, NIV). Jonah went on to lead the entire corrupt city of Nineveh back to God.

The demon-possessed man became a walking testimony of Jesus' miraculous healing power. *He went all through the town proclaiming the great things Jesus had done for him* (Luke 8:39).

Westley was left for dead in the "pit of despair." No longer able to rely on his physical stamina and expert fencing skills, he saved Princess Buttercup from the evil Prince Humperdinck by using his intellect.

Our lives are so full of busyness and distraction that sometimes the quiet stillness of the pit is exactly where we need to be in order to hear the still, small voice. God may be using this opportunity to get our full and undivided attention. When we look up from the pit, our eyes are no longer on our circumstances or surroundings, but on the loving face of our Heavenly Father. God uses our time in the pit to soften our hearts toward Him so that He can reshape them to look more like His.

Remember the height from which you have fallen! Repent and do the things you did at first. If you do not repent, I will come and remove your lampstand from its place (Revelation 2:5, NIV).

At times I might shut up the heavens so that no rain falls, or command grasshoppers to devour your crops, or send plagues among you. Then if my people who are called by my name will humble themselves and pray and seek my face and turn from their wicked ways, I will hear from heaven and will forgive their sins and restore their land (2 Chronicles 7:13-14).

Do not gloat over me my enemy! Though I have fallen, I will rise. Though I sit in darkness, the Lord will be my light (Micah 7:8, NIV).

Turn your eyes upon Jesus, look full in His wonderful face, and the things of earth will grow strangely dim in the light of His glory and grace.[5]

---

[5] Lemmel, Helen H. Turn Your Eyes Upon Jesus, 1922. Public domain.

Identifying Spiritual Strongholds

> *Put on all of God's armor so that you will be able to
> stand firm against all strategies of the devil. For we are not
> fighting against flesh-and-blood enemies, but against evil rulers
> and authorities of the unseen world, against mighty powers in
> this dark world, and against evil spirits in the heavenly places*
> (Ephesians 6:11-12).

> *Stay alert! Watch out for your great enemy, the devil. He
> prowls around like a roaring lion, looking for someone to
> devour. Stand firm against him, and be strong in your faith*
> (I Peter 5:8-9).

While every pit has similar components, the specific "décor" is highly tailored to the individual in the form of strongholds. Don't let the word "stronghold" scare you away. It is merely anything that has a "strong hold" on us, keeping us from enjoying freedom and victory in our lives. The enemy knows exactly where we are most vulnerable and will attempt to use those areas to keep us chained and miserable in our pit.

While Satan may be crafty, he is not very creative. He often uses variations of the same strongholds: depression, anxiety, jealousy, and relational discord to shake our faith and take our focus off of God.

Depression

From the depths of despair, O Lord, I call for your help. Hear my cry, O Lord. Pay attention to my prayer
(Psalm 130:1-2).

Depression is usually brought on by an overwhelming feeling of despair, the fading of all hope or confidence. It causes us to feel so completely overwhelmed by darkness that we can see nothing but our own misery. We see no reason to get out of bed in the morning because depression gives us the illusion that we have nothing to look forward to and nothing to live for.

There is a common misconception that depression should not affect Christ followers and is a sure sign of not being "spiritual" enough. There's one problem with that theory: it's not Biblical.

King David was "a man after God's own heart" (I Samuel 13:14), yet he consistently struggled with very serious bouts of depression. The *Psalms* are a collection of David's most private thoughts and feelings. Though he wrote many beautiful songs of praise, he wrote just as often of his experiences with intense grief and crippling despair.

The great prophet, Elijah, came to such a dark point in his ministry that he wanted to die. He actually sat down under a tree and prayed, "I have had enough, Lord. Take my life" (I Kings 19:4, NIV).

Abraham was called "righteous" by the Almighty God Himself (Genesis 15:6), yet even *he* is quoted as saying, "What good are all your blessings when I don't even have a son?" (Genesis 15: 2). As we discussed earlier, Hannah cried bitterly in deep anguish and became so distraught that she could not eat (I Samuel 1:7, 10).

Even Jesus, in anticipation of the cross, had a brief encounter with depression. The Bible says that as He entered the Garden of Gethsemane, Jesus became "anguished and distressed" (Matthew 6:37). He told his closest friends, "My soul is crushed with grief to the point of death" (Matthew 6:38).

And then there was Job. *Groan.* You knew it was coming, didn't you? After all, there can't be a candid discussion about depression from a Biblical perspective without mentioning Job.

When I was in my own pit of despair – I mean really at rock bottom here – a family member told me to read the Book of Job. She might as well have slapped me across the face. Knowing the depth of the depression I was in, she thought it would be a *good* idea to have me read the most notoriously depressing book in the whole Bible? I thought, *"Seriously?* Do you *want* me to kill myself?" At least the depressing parts in the Book of Psalm are nicely sandwiched in with songs of praise, worship, and encouragement. Job is forty-two chapters of gut-wrenching pain and suffering.

For those of you who are not familiar with the saga of Job, it is the story of a wealthy and devoted man of God who is suddenly hit with overwhelming loss. The Book of Job begins with a conversation between God and Satan in which God brags on Job's character.

Have you noticed my servant Job? He is the finest man in all the earth. He is blameless – a man of complete integrity. He fears God and stays away from evil." Satan replied to the Lord, "Yes, but Job has good reason to fear God. You have always put a wall of protection around him and his home and his property. You have made him prosper in everything he does. Look how rich he is! But reach out and take away everything he has and he will surely curse you to your face! (Job 1:8-11).

God accepts this challenge in order to prove Job's faithfulness. One by one, all of Job's blessings are stripped away: his livestock, camels, servants and children, all in a matter of a few hours. Job was understandably devastated, yet he still fell to his knees to worship God. *Naked I came from my mother's womb and naked I will depart. The Lord gave and the Lord has taken away. Blessed be the name of the Lord* (Job 1:21, NIV).

Things go from bad to worse as God then allows Satan to strike Job with boils from head to foot. Job's wife tells him to curse God and die, and his closest friends accuse him of having brought this on himself through hidden sin in his life.

It is important to remember that Job was not privy to the conversations between God and Satan, so Job has no idea why God is allowing these catastrophes to keep happening. All he knows is that he feels picked on. Hurt. Betrayed. Angry. In ultimate despair, Job cries out to God:

I wish he would crush me. I wish he would reach out his hand and kill me (Job 6:9).

I would rather be strangled – rather die than suffer like this. I hate my life and don't want to go on living. Oh, leave me alone for my few remaining days (Job 7:15).

Why won't you leave me alone, at least long enough for me to swallow! If I have sinned, what have I done to you, O watcher of all humanity? Why make me your target? Am I a burden to you? (Job 7:19-20).

My days are over. My hopes have disappeared. My heart's desires are broken (Job 17:11).

Not exactly the kind of stuff you find in greeting cards. But can you relate? I know I can. I had lost all hope in ever having a baby. I had determined that it was something that would happen to everyone else who even had a fleeting desire to procreate, but it was never going to happen to me. Not now. Not ever.

On the outside I would smile and nod when people said I would get pregnant eventually, just to wait and be patient. On the inside I was shaking my head and resisting the urge to slap the happy right out of them. Who were they kidding? It's clearly not meant for me to be a parent, just like my well-meaning friend had already pointed out.

I was not well in any sense of the word. Nathan did his best to comfort me but when I wasn't "better" in a few days, he threw his hands up. He did not know how to deal with me in this state of hopelessness, so he chose not to deal with me at all. He made himself scarce on nights and weekends, leaving me alone with my despair.

It was a Saturday morning in mid-December. The despair and depression had taken over to the point of crippling me. I had not eaten, showered, brushed my hair or changed out of the same raggedy sweats in days. Like David, I was *worn out from groaning; all night long I flood my bed with weeping and drench my couch with tears* (Psalm 6:6, NIV).

I remember opening the medicine cabinet and taking a mental inventory of what I saw: old prescription for Valium from last year's surgery, a few Darvocet, cold medicine, and a full bottle of aspirin. I had a sudden urge to dump every bottle I could find into a colorful pile and swallow every pill until I couldn't feel the pain anymore. My destructive thoughts frightened me. I slammed the cabinet shut and ran back to bed, praying that God would just *take* me so I wouldn't have to spend another day in this miserable existence.

Just as I pulled the covers back over my head, the doorbell rang. Probably a door-to-door salesperson, I told myself. I had absolutely no intention of getting out of bed. Ding-dong. Ding-dong. DIIINGGGG.....DOOONNNG. Then there was knocking. Someone was very determined, that's all I knew. Annoyed, I threw back the covers and stormed to the front door, flung it open and prepared to give the person standing there a piece of my mind.

Staring back at me was my best friend from high school, Kelly. She had moved 300 miles away two years earlier to pursue her career and I had missed her terribly. I didn't want to burden her with what was going on because I knew she would worry, being so far away and unable to do anything. I was absolutely humiliated that she had to see me like this.

"Oh, Kel..." It was as if a dam inside of me had broken, letting out a flood of emotions that I had been unable to release before that moment. I began to sob uncontrollably, collapsing in the dark entryway as she knelt to wrap her arms around me and smooth my stringy hair with her hands. She let me cry until every ounce of energy within me was exhausted, then did something that I believe saved my life.

"Come on, get up," she said firmly, helping me to my feet. She held me at arms length and looked me over.

"Oh no, girl. You're not doing this anymore. Let's get you ready. I've got to get you out of this house."

The thought of functioning like a normal human being was overwhelming. I started to cry again as she led me by the arm to the master bathroom and turned on the shower. She found my hair brush and began to untangle my hair in long, smooth strokes.

"How did you know?" I managed to ask.

Nathan had called her in desperation, knowing that I wouldn't, and asked for her help.

I showered for the first time in days while Kelly went through my closet and picked out something for me to wear. I was still so emotionally numb that I felt as if I were doing everything in slow motion. Kelly stood outside the door, encouraging me to take my time but to get it done.

I did not want to leave the house but had very little fight left in me. All I could do in the way of a protest was whimper as Kelly put my shoes on and led me to the front door by the shoulders.

The sun felt warm on my face and awakened a part of me that I thought was gone forever. I closed my eyes and took a deep breath of the cool December air, filled with smells of chimney smoke and pine trees. I heard children laughing at the playground across the street.

With each breath I felt more and more alive. It was exhilarating and frightening at the same time. If I actually enjoyed life again would that mean I was betraying the memory of the baby I had lost? Would it mean I didn't care? What kind of mother smiles and laughs less than a month after the loss of a child? How could I possibly be worthy of another baby if I just went on with my life like nothing happened? These mental onslaughts from the enemy caused me to hang my head with shame and I began to cry again. Kelly lifted my chin with her hand.

"Clair, God doesn't want you to hurt like this anymore. He wants to heal your heart. Life is still going on all around you and you can choose to be a part of it or you can continue to check out. You are not going to check out any more. Not on my watch. Enough is enough."

As she pulled into the TCBY® parking lot, she laid her hand on mine and asked God to heal my heart from this loss, to heal my emotions from this debilitating depression and to heal my spirit, which had taken a beating by the enemy. She prayed for peace that passes all understanding to flow through me and for God to be that friend that sticks closer than a brother when I felt lonely and sad. Instantly the dark cloud that had been hovering over my spirit lifted. I felt as if a huge weight had been lifted off of me and I could breathe again.

We laughed – actually laughed – over white chocolate mousse yogurt with chocolate chip cookie dough and splurged on waffle cones with sprinkles. Something so simple made a world of difference for me. Kelly was my saving grace that day. I needed to hear the truth spoken in love and God had sent her to do just that.

Come quickly, Lord, and answer me, for my depression deepens. Don't turn away from me, or I will die (Psalm 143:7).

Why am I discouraged? Why is my heart so sad? I will put my hope in God! I will praise him again – my Savior and my God! (Psalm 42:5).

You keep track of all my sorrows. You have collected all my tears in your bottle. You have recorded each one in your book (Psalm 56:8).

The Lord is close to the brokenhearted; he rescues those whose spirits are crushed (Psalm 34:18).

Those who plant in tears will harvest with shouts of joy (Psalm 126:5).

Anxiety

I...was troubled in spirit and the visions that passed through my mind disturbed me (Daniel 7:15, NIV).

Anxiety is a self-imposed prison. Racing thoughts lead to panic. An overwhelming feeling of losing control causes the room to spin and leaves you disoriented. A vague dread looms like an ominous storm cloud, though dread of *what* exactly you can't seem to figure out. Obsessive worrying leaves you incapacitated, paralyzed by fear of the unknown until the fear becomes bigger than the problem itself. You're restless, staring at the ceiling night after night while everyone else is sleeping soundly. Stress levels are high and tolerance levels are low. You feel like a hamster in a cage, spinning your wheels but going nowhere for fear that if you slow down, even for a moment, you'll be forced to face the uncertainties that lie ahead.

Worry and stress are not unique to the 21st century. King Nebuchadnezzar was one of the most powerful leaders of his time, yet in the midst of "comfort and prosperity," he became frightened with visions of a bleak future (Daniel 4:4-26). Likewise, it wasn't the lions den that terrified the great prophet Daniel, it was his thoughts (Daniel 4:19).

Jesus certainly had plenty to say on the subject. *Can all your worries add a single moment to your life?* (Matthew 6:27, NIV). *Give your entire attention to what God is doing right now, and don't get worked up about what may or may not happen tomorrow. God will help you deal with whatever hard things come up when the time comes* (Matthew 6:34, The Message). Later on, Jesus tells Martha, the 'hostess with the mostess,' "Martha, dear Martha...you're getting yourself worked up over nothing (Luke 10:41, The Message). Yet even Jesus was under so much stress before his crucifixion at the thought of being separated from his Father that "his sweat fell to the ground like great drops of blood" (Luke 22:44).

Anxiety is counterproductive because it does not change or solve anything. It only robs us of today by draining our energy. Rather than meditating on God's word and His promises, we meditate on our own thoughts and feelings, which are unreliable and not always based on truth.

Fertility issues are a source of great anxiety for many women. Fear of all of the unknowns can be overwhelming. Fear of more disappointment or loss. Fear of making the wrong choice when it comes to infertility options. Fear of financial issues caused by mounting medical bills. Fear that relationships may not survive the pressure and strain caused by infertility or miscarriage. Even being around other pregnant women can be the source of great angst. At least it certainly was for me.

My relationship with Jennifer had remained friendly but strained. It was much easier talking to her on the phone because I was not face-to-face with her "baby bump." We generally avoided discussions about her pregnancy unless I brought it up, which I forced myself to do from time to time.

Panic set in as I realized I should be planning a baby shower for Jennifer. After all, I was her best friend. It would be expected. Just the thought of sitting next to her with her big, round belly and glowing smile, recording each baby gift as she opened it, and trying to guess in toilet paper squares just how big her growing belly was made me want to put my head between my knees and breathe deeply into a paper bag. Nevertheless, I was determined to do it. Surely I could put aside my own grief for a few hours to celebrate the impending arrival of my best friend's first baby. Yet as the shower date grew closer, I began to grow more and more anxious.

I was pushing a shopping cart in the middle of Wal-Mart when I started thinking about the baby shower. All of a sudden I felt as if I were in a tunnel. My hearing became muffled as if I had cotton balls stuffed in my ears. All I could hear was my own heart beating, the methodical *thud-thud-thud* growing faster and louder. Everything around me looked like blurry colors and shapes. Although I was sweating profusely, my teeth were chattering like I was sitting in the middle of a snowstorm in a bikini. The walls seemed to be closing in around me. I needed to get out of there...now.

I left the shopping cart, full of groceries, in the middle of an aisle and made my way to the front of the store, holding onto anything I could get my hands on to steady myself.

"Ma'am? Ma'am, are you O.K.?"

I was only vaguely aware of the woman in the blue vest as I blew right past her, leaving behind shopping carts and the larger than life yellow smiley faces that seemed to be laughing at me. I stumbled through the automatic double doors onto the sidewalk outside and forced myself to breathe. The fresh air burned my lungs and I felt so dizzy I thought I might fall down. I bent over and gripped my knees for support as I closed my eyes and managed to collect my thoughts enough to murmur a short prayer asking God to help me find my car. I just wanted to go home and cry.

As the shower date grew closer, these episodes began to occur more and more frequently. They would arise seemingly out of nowhere: while I was driving, in the middle of my work day, while exercising. There was no rhyme or reason to them, but they were definitely interfering with my life to the point where I needed some help.

My family doctor believed I was suffering from severe anxiety that was manifesting itself in the form of panic attacks.

"So I'm crazy." There was a hint of irritation in my voice.

"No, you're not crazy. You have been through a lot and you need to give yourself some time to heal." The doctor scribbled something on a prescription pad. "And you should really think twice about going to this shower. I think it's a bad idea."

Whatever. That was easier said than done. You don't just miss your best friend's baby shower. No matter what. I was a tough woman and I had been through far worse things. Yet when the day came, I couldn't do it. More guilt piled on top of what had already consumed me. It was a vicious cycle. Anxiety led to guilt, which led to more anxiety. It was no way to live. That's all I knew for sure.

God offers the only lasting antidote for anxiety: His peace. Jesus said, "I am leaving you with a gift – peace of mind and heart. And the peace I give is a gift the world cannot give. So don't be troubled or afraid" (John 14:27). In his letter to the Philippians, Paul writes, "Don't worry about anything; instead, pray about everything. Tell God what you need, and thank him for all he has done. Then you will experience God's peace, which exceeds anything we can understand. His peace will guard your hearts and minds as you live in Christ Jesus" (Philippians 4:6-7). *His* peace: a peace neither found in the absence of problems nor in the "power of positive thinking" that the world promotes. It is a place of rest in knowing that God is in control and He is bigger than any problem we face. *Nothing* is too difficult for Him (Jeremiah 32:17). Not broken relationships, not finances, not unstable emotions, and certainly not infertility.

Search me, O God, and know my heart;
test me and know my anxious thoughts (Psalm 139:23).

The Lord is my light and my salvation –
So why should I be afraid?
The Lord is my fortress, protecting me from danger,
So why should I tremble? (Psalm 27:1).

Give your burdens to the Lord,
and he will take care of you.
He will not permit the godly to slip and fall (Psalm 55:22).

When doubts filled my mind,
your comfort gave me renewed hope and cheer (Psalm 94:19).

When I am overwhelmed, you alone know the way I should turn
(Psalm 142:3).

The Lord helps the fallen and lifts those bent beneath their loads
(Psalm 145:14).

Jealousy

> *Anger is cruel, and wrath is like a flood,*
> *but jealousy is even more dangerous* (Proverbs 27:4).

> *O beware of jealousy! It is the green-eyed monster that*
> *doth mock the meat it feeds upon*
> (William Shakespeare, *Othello*, Act III, Scene iii).

Jealousy has been rearing its ugly head since the beginning of time. The first recorded homicide was a result of intense jealousy that had grown into hatred. Cain could not stand that his brother, Abel, had something Cain so desperately wanted – God's favor (Genesis 4:2-5). All Cain had to do was heed God's instructions on how to get his heart in the right place so that he, too, could also experience favor. Instead, Cain eliminates his competition by killing Abel (Genesis 4:8).

After David's crushing defeat of Goliath, King Saul considered David to be invaluable, the greatest warrior in his kingdom (I Samuel 18:2, 5). But Saul's admiration quickly turned to jealousy whenever the people began to see David as a better warrior than Saul.

> *[W]omen from all the towns of Israel came out to meet King Saul. They sang and danced for joy with tambourines and cymbals. This was their song: "Saul has killed his thousands, and David his ten thousands!" This made Saul very angry. "What's this?" he said. "They credit David with ten thousands and me with only thousands. Next they'll be making him their king!" So from that time on Saul kept a jealous eye on David* (I Samuel 18:6-9).

Saul's jealousy soon turned to intense hatred and he made numerous attempts to kill David, as recorded throughout the rest of I Samuel. In the middle of one of his rampages, Saul even tried to kill his own son, Jonathan (I Samuel 20:33). It just goes to show how we can become so blind with jealousy that we don't even realize we are not only hurting those closest to us, but ourselves as well. Saul's jealousy toward David had caused Saul to forget everything else that was important to him. Both his kingdom and his family paid the price. *For jealousy and selfishness are not God's kind of wisdom. Such things are earthly, unspiritual and demonic. For wherever there is jealousy and selfish ambition, there you will find disorder and evil of every kind* (James 3:14-16).

It became more and more difficult for me to be around pregnant women or new mothers. Mother's Day rolled around and I could not even bring myself to go to church. Just the thought of sitting through a sermon on the joys of motherhood and how *her children rise up and call her blessed* (Proverbs 31:28) with a sanctuary full of women wearing corsages and holding little ones made me want to gag. I had decided they were all set on making me miserable, rubbing it in my face that they had a baby and I did not. Complicating the matter was that my closest friend was, in fact, still growing more and more pregnant with each passing week.

With her first trimester safely behind her, Jennifer called to tell me that she and Brian would be announcing her pregnancy to our Sunday School Class in the upcoming weekend.

"Great," I scowled. "Thanks for telling me. Won't be there."

I just couldn't stand the thought of everyone smiling and congratulating Jennifer when I wanted them to be doing the same for me. They *would have* if I hadn't lost the baby. Our due dates had been only two weeks apart and we had planned on announcing our pregnancies together. Now Jennifer was still in the "pregnant club" and I had been cruelly excommunicated.

I made the mistake of calling Jennifer right after one of my doctor appointments following the miscarriage. There was complete silence on the other end of the phone as I ranted and raved about all the "happy pregnant people" in the lobby and how sick to death I was of being surrounded by them everywhere I went.

"*What*? What's wrong?" I spouted off, half irritated that she hadn't agreed with me.

"It's just that...when you talk about 'happy pregnant people,' you're talking about *me*, Clair. Only I feel like I can't be happy about this pregnancy with you. You're my best friend and I hate that you are going through so much, but you make me feel guilty for being pregnant."

Oh wow. I hadn't even thought of that. I wanted to be happy for Jennifer. I really did. At any other time in my life it would have been a no-brainer, but I was too wrapped up in jealousy and self-pity at the moment and didn't know quite how to dig myself out of it. I wasn't pregnant anymore...and I didn't want *her* to be either. I couldn't stand the sight of my own best friend because she had something that I had wanted so much. I just wanted things to go back to the way they were.

The only thing I knew to do was to distance myself from Jennifer so she wouldn't have to feel guilty around *me* and I wouldn't have to feel jealous of *her*. I thought that was the best thing for both of us – especially for *her* since I was such a terrible friend.

The day Jennifer called to tell me she had just delivered a healthy baby boy was bitter sweet. I slid down the wall next to the phone until I was sitting on the floor, tears filling my eyes. Happy tears for her, as the moment she had been waiting for all these months was finally here; bitter tears for myself, knowing I should have been days away from delivering my own child. But this was *her* moment. Not mine.

"Can I come see you...and the baby?" I knew I had not been a very good friend and Jennifer had every right to say "no," but I missed her so much and this was one of the most important moments of her life. I wanted to be there and at least *try* to share that with her.

"Of course." There was gentleness and understanding in Jennifer's voice. She knew this was hard for me but she wanted – *needed* – me to get over myself and be a friend. Her *best* friend. *Oh, God. Heal my heart and give me the strength that I need. I can't do this without you.*

I called my florist, ordered an arrangement with daisies (Jennifer's favorite), and stopped to pick it up on the way to the hospital. My heart was pounding and my mind racing in a million different directions. *Do I think I can hold the baby? What if she tries to hand him to me and I know I'm going to freak out? How can I get out of it without hurting her feelings?*

What's my exit strategy if I feel a meltdown coming on? There were too many variables; too many things to think about.

I paused outside Jennifer's hospital room and took a deep breath, exhaling into a big smile as I walked into the room. Jennifer was cradling a tiny bundle while Brian sat next to her. I added my flowers to the growing collection on the windowsill and took a seat next to Jennifer, staring at the round, pink face with a white stocking cap.

"Oh, Jen. He's beautiful." It was hard to imagine that just the day before this little guy was still living inside of her.

Jennifer's blue eyes were studying me, searching for clues as to what I may be thinking or feeling.

"Do you want to hold him?" she asked, taking a chance.

Good question. *Did* I?

"You don't have to," she quickly added.

"No. I, uh...I want to," the words coming out of my mouth surprised even me.

She carefully shifted the swaddled baby boy into my arms. He absolutely took my breath away. I couldn't stop staring at him. He was so peaceful, so content. His tiny fingers wrapped around my thumb and I was absolutely awestruck. So this is what it would have felt like to be a mommy. Maybe if Jennifer could just share him with me, just sometimes, my broken heart could slowly begin to heal.

For love is as strong as death and jealousy as cruel as the grave
(Song of Songs 8:6, NKJV).

Love is not jealous (I Corinthians 13:4).

Let us not...be jealous of one another (Galatians 5:26).

71

Relational Issues

Be happy with those who are happy,
and weep with those who weep (Romans 12:15).

Infertility and miscarriage can wreak havoc on the relationships in our lives. When emotions run high, it's easy to lash out on the people closest to us. Marriages suffer when sex becomes more of a methodical science experiment than a spontaneous expression of love. It becomes difficult to maintain a normal relationship with friends or family members who are so fertile that their husbands just have to *look* at them when they're ovulating and they become pregnant. Especially for those of us who are on prescription fertility drugs, taking our temperature, playing Twister in the bedroom, shoving pillows under our hips to keep everything "in"... and still not getting anywhere.

A great example of how infertility affects relationships is found in the saga of the Bible's most famous love triangle: Jacob, Rachel and Leah. This whole situation was messed up from the beginning. Leah and Rachel were the original *Desperate Housewives*. See for yourself in Genesis 29-30. It is a sordid, twisted tale of sex, lies and back-stabbing.

Here's the abbreviated version: Jacob works seven years for Rachel and Leah's father, Laban, in exchange for Rachel's hand in marriage. Only Laban pulls a switcheroo on Jacob on the long-awaited wedding day and the veiled woman at the altar is actually Leah (inferred in Genesis 29:17 as the older, less attractive sister)! Laban tells Jacob if he wants Rachel, he will have to work another seven years (v. 26-27). Talk about blackmail.

Jacob loved Rachel much more than Leah (v. 30), although he apparently didn't mind sleeping with Leah because she soon began having his babies, one after another, until she had given him four sons (v. 32-35). But Rachel could not get pregnant (v. 31).

> *"When Rachel saw that she wasn't having any children for Jacob, she became jealous of her sister. She pleaded with Jacob, 'Give me children, or I'll die!' Then Jacob became furious with Rachel. 'Am I God?' he asked. 'He's the one who has kept you from having children!'"*
> (Genesis 30:1-2).

Rather than giving God her pain, jealousy, and anger over her inability to conceive, Rachel let it consume her to the point where she could no longer think clearly. God was no longer a priority. Jacob's love and adoration was no longer enough. This tunnel vision turned into a relational train wreck as first Rachel, then Leah, offer their maids to Jacob as wives in a twisted competition fueled by selfishness to "one up" each other.

You may have thought of some of your own strained relationships when you read the story of Rachel and Leah. In my case, I let my desire to have a baby consume me. It was more important than my relationship with God, my husband, friends, family, and church. I let the enemy isolate me from my closest alliances, especially other believers.

I remained angry at God, but forced myself to have quiet time on occasion because I was "supposed to." I flipped open to the Book of Romans one morning and what I read made me so angry at God that I wanted to hurl my Bible across the room: *[W]e also rejoice in our sufferings, because we know that suffering produces perseverance; perseverance, character; and character, hope* (Romans 5:3-4, NIV).

I had read that verse dozens of times before when the planets were in perfect alignment and the sun was shining and birds were chirping. Sure, it was easy to agree with that under perfect circumstances, but in the midst of the storms of "suffering" it just made me *mad*. In my own limited mind, I already had enough "character" to single-handedly cast a thirty-minute sitcom. I certainly did not need any more of it. I blamed God for picking on me and leaving me to rot in the depths of my pit. What kind of Father abandons His child when she is hurting the most?

I let envy and selfishness lead to strife in my relationship with Jennifer, one of my best friends who had what I so desperately wanted. I had once picked up the phone to call her with anything and everything I needed to talk about. Now, full of guilt and feeling like the worst friend *ever*, I hesitated. I used the new baby as an excuse, not wanting to wake either of them or telling myself Jennifer had her hands full as it was.

But it was my relationship with Nathan that took the biggest hit. Tragedy can do one of two things to a marriage: it can bring you closer together or it can tear you apart if you are unable or unwilling to work through it. That's exactly what happened to us. Both Nathan and I had suffered incredible losses and hurt before we came together – losses that were stuffed down deep inside where no one else could see them. Our marriage had been hanging on by a thread for years. The miscarriages took what little remained and left it even more frayed and weak.

Life slowly but surely started to get back to normal – as normal as life can be anyway. Nathan and I did our best to put on a happy face for everyone else while ignoring the vast cavern that had grown in between us. The loss of the baby had only created more distance. We lived very separate lives while sharing the same address.

Three months later, when I discovered I was pregnant again, Jennifer was the only one who knew about it. I did not want to deal with another less than enthusiastic reception from Nathan and I honestly did not even know if I *wanted* to be pregnant. At one time it seemed like a good idea, but the more I thought about it, the more I realized that a baby would not fix our broken marriage. We would just be bringing an innocent child into the mix and the three of us would end up more hurt in the long run. God must have agreed because right before my first doctor appointment, I began to bleed again. Another loss. Only this time I needed a D&C.

"I'm sorry, Clair. I really am," Nathan said over the phone when I asked if he could go with me to the procedure. "But I have a meeting at work that I really shouldn't miss unless you just absolutely need me there."

I had a terrible fear of confrontation, so although I felt abandoned by Nathan after the *first* miscarriage and was angry that he put his job before me after the *second* one, I said nothing. I just froze him out until I was no longer angry – just indifferent toward him. I simply did not care anymore.

Nathan had deep hurts from his own childhood and adolescence that were just as painful as my own. What we did not realize at the time is that the things we kept hidden were the things that had the deepest hold on us. Bitterness and resentment had taken root long before we ever met, producing a crop of displaced anger that we took out on each other.

Nathan and I were barely more than polite strangers living under the same roof. There was no animosity between us, just vague indifference. The topic of separation and divorce was one we dared not speak of, yet it was obvious that it had crossed each of our minds.

The crazy thing is that we were both Christians. We both knew who God was. We read the Bible. We were active in our church. We had both been baptized. We prayed before meals and bed. What is *sad* is that we thought that was enough. God remained an intimate stranger. We knew a lot *about* Him, just like we knew a lot about famous politicians or sports figures, but we did not have a personal relationship with Him. He remained at arms length, distant and aloof. That wasn't *His* choice. It was *ours*. I don't even think it was a *conscious* choice on our part. We just didn't know any different.

Issues that we kept buried, though just below the surface, slowly began to emerge. Lines were crossed. Deception and secrets crept in. Promises were broken. Wounds remained open and festering despite our best efforts to slap a band-aid over them. Our relationship was beyond repair. It was really over.

Eight and a half years into our marriage, I found myself in a one-bedroom apartment, surrounded by boxes and the smells of fresh paint and new carpet.

"How much longer do I have to hurt, Lord?" I asked aloud.

I had failed at motherhood, friendship and now marriage.

"What more do you *want* from me?" I screamed out loud, "Why are you doing this? What have I done to you?"

But my questions just reverberated off the sterile walls. I sat in the living room floor that first night alone with my head in my hands and cried until I couldn't cry anymore. I was totally and completely broken. I had never felt so alone in my entire life and I had no idea how everything was going to work out.

Don't just pretend to love others. Really love them (Romans 12:9).

How wonderful and pleasant it is when brothers live together in harmony! (Psalm 133:1).

Get rid of all bitterness, rage, anger, harsh words, and slander, as well as all types of evil behavior. Instead, be kind to each other, tenderhearted, forgiving one another, just as God through Christ has forgiven you (Ephesians 4:31-32).

Love is patient and kind. Love is not jealous or boastful or proud or rude. It does not demand its own way. It is not irritable, and it keeps no record of being wronged. It does not rejoice about injustice but rejoices when the truth wins out. Love never gives up, never loses faith, is always hopeful, and endures through every circumstance (1 Corinthians 13:4-7).

Chapter 4: The Road to Healing and Restoration

I will repay you for the years the locusts have eaten
(Joel 2:25, NIV).

I personally don't have anything against locusts. Call me crazy, but I think they are beautiful creatures with their hues of emerald green and the intricate details on their wings. One of the things I remember about summers in West Texas is the sound of locusts at dusk. It's one of the things I miss about home.

The Israelites in the Old Testament had a completely different take on locusts. They were symbols of destruction and loss. Crops which had taken years of blood, sweat, and tears could be destroyed in a matter of hours as swarms of locusts took one tiny bite at a time. *What the locust swarm has left the great locusts have eaten; what the great locusts have left the young locusts have eaten; what the young locusts have left other locusts have eaten* (Joel 1:4, NIV).

It doesn't take a background in agriculture to understand how the words of the prophet Joel still apply. Have you ever felt like you were being picked apart by one situation, crisis, or relationship after another? I have. What was left of my confidence and self-esteem after events from my past was picked at by my ex-husband. What was left of my hope was snatched away by the miscarriages and so on until all that was left, despite years of being rooted in faith as a Christ-follower, was a raw skeleton of my former self. I felt as if I had nothing else to give and nothing else that could be taken from me. Yet God promises to restore the locust years.

My stint in "the pit" had forced me to look up. But *now* what? After all, I was still mad! The first thing God did to minister to my spirit was show me that I had not dealt with many of my hurts, and if I wanted to get over being mad there were some things I needed to work through.

I had ignored deep emotional wounds and a broken spirit for so long that wrong ways of thinking, resentment, and unforgiveness had taken root, producing the fruit of bitterness. It had grown rampant like spiritual cancer, poisoning everything I said and everything I did. It was hard to admit, but it was the truth, and confessing it was the very first step toward healing. Step one of many. *Then you will know the truth and the truth will set you free* (John 8:32, NIV).

The path toward healing is not an easy road to follow. It's like entering a marathon when all you really want to do is jog around the block and call it a day. Some of us are so eager to hurry along the process that we invest in a good pair of running shoes, determined to sprint through the valleys, up the winding hills until we reach the very top of the hill where an imaginary flag is staked in the ground. It waves to us, beckoning, and as we draw closer we can make out the words "The End".

The end to our pain. The end to our sorrow. The end to disappointment and discouragement. We long for God to hold our head in His hands and erase all of these things like a clean sweep across a chalkboard, and we want it done as quickly and painlessly as possible.

Our society is not known for its patience. Instant gratification is something we all have grown accustomed to. I'll be the first to admit I have approached God on more than one occasion with this mindset and expected Him to have the same time measurements and limitations that I do. As far as healing was concerned, I tried to be a sprinter. I didn't want to take the time to work on it gradually. I wanted results *now*. Let me save you some time before you go out looking for a good pair of running shoes to race through your own healing. *You cannot undo something in a day that has taken months or even years to accumulate.* God will see you through in His own gentle way, which far exceeds anything you could ever accomplish on your own.

Healing is as much work as physical exercise. Every January 1st, local gyms are packed with the "good intentions crowd" - those who have made New Year's resolutions to improve their health or physical attractiveness through exercise and, most of the time, diet. Personal trainers are booked with back-to-back appointments of those who want to have a chiseled physique by spring break.

Many of the "good intentions crowd" truly *intend* to be faithful to their exercise routine and are feeling relatively nourished on lettuce, tofu and black coffee until about January 5th. When their stomachs still do not resemble a washboard and there is no sign of improvement for the hail damage on the backs of their thighs, a large percentage of them drop out. Why? There is no instant gratification in diet and exercise.

So many people miss out on the rewards of having achieved physical fitness. Not only do the muscles look toned and well defined, but energy levels increase. Sleep patterns stabilize. Life is seen in a whole new light when the body is in maximum shape. Those who are willing to put in the time, sweat, and toil will reap the rewards. Those who are *not*, on the other hand, are stuck with the unsettling feeling of being less than fit.

Just like exercise, it takes time, sweat, and toil to work through emotional healing. It involves allowing yourself to be totally vulnerable again, sometimes reliving the original trauma and breaking open old wounds in order to *feel* again. If you've grown accustomed to being numb, this can be very uncomfortable and upsetting.

When I first began my own healing process, I felt like my heart had been turned inside out, exposed and raw. It was like having a broken bone that had not healed correctly. I knew it didn't look or feel right, but I had grown comfortable with the way it was. I didn't want to go through the pain of having it broken again, not to mention the process of being immobile while it healed properly.

I chose to ignore my emotional wounds for far too long. Scar tissue had formed around them, like uneven knots protruding out from a limb. In the beginning, it would only throb on occasion – nothing that a little self-medication couldn't fix. Over time, the throb progressed to a sharp, searing pain that ran all the way through my body until I could not stand it any longer. The pain was too great to keep ignoring it. It was going to continue to make its presence known until I dealt with the underlying problem.

In order to truly heal and experience genuine freedom, I had to be willing to allow Jesus to chisel away at the scars and "re-break" some things within me so He could set them properly. By not doing things right the first time, I ended up dealing with the pain a lot longer than I needed to.

Broken, exhausted, and feeling completely defeated, I managed to humbly ask Him for help. I needed healing and I knew only Jesus could help me. He was there, waiting and willing, the entire time. All I had to do was invite Him into the broken places of my heart; places I never would have visited again had He not gone back there with me. Layer after layer began to peel away until nothing was left but *me* in all of my emotional and spiritual nakedness before Him. It was scary being that vulnerable, even to Jesus. "Do you trust me?" I could hear him gently ask.

"Yes, Lord," I answered. "I trust you."

Did it happen overnight? Oh, goodness, no. I had a lot of junk to work through and I wanted to do it right this time so I wouldn't have to keep going back there. Was it painful? Yes. Excruciating, in fact. But was it worth it? Absolutely. The Son has set me free and I am free indeed (John 8:36)!

> *I waited patiently for the Lord; he turned to me and heard my cry. He lifted me out of the slimy pit, out of the mud and mire; he set my feet on a rock and gave me a firm place to stand. He put a new song in my mouth, a hymn of praise to our God* (Psalm 40:1-3, NIV).

> *O Lord, my God, I called to you for help and you healed me* (Psalm 30:2, NIV).

Weeping may last for the night, but joy comes in the morning! (Psalm 30:5, NIV).

[W]herever the Spirit of the Lord is, there is freedom (2 Corinthians 3:17).

(Just Like) Starting Over

For the first couple of weeks on my own, I did little more than go through the motions of life. I was so numb that someone could have stabbed me repeatedly with a fork and I wouldn't have flinched. My thinking was cloudy and my emotions were raw. I missed Nathan in some ways and was so angry with him in others. I was hurt by the people I thought would stand by me but *didn't* and pleasantly surprised by the people I least expected to be there for me yet *were*. I was grief-stricken; mourning over the death of my marriage, the dreams that went with it, and the thought of losing an extended family that I had grown to love very much. I wanted to scream at the top of my lungs until I couldn't scream anymore. I wanted to hit something. I wanted to *feel* again.

I had just finished my first year of law school at Texas Tech when Nathan and I separated. When word got out that I was going through a divorce, my wonderful friends and classmates whom I had known for less than a year rallied around me. One friend in particular knew exactly what I was going through. His name was Victor Rivera. Victor and I met during the first week of law school and were in the same section, which meant we had every class together for the entire first year. We were destined to be friends from the very start.

During the first week of school, the Board of Legal Examiners required all law students to be fingerprinted in order to complete background checks. When it was my turn, I noticed the people in charge of fingerprinting were doing them all wrong. I had done quite a bit of fingerprinting as a probation officer and had been through enough training to know that smudged prints would not be accepted by the State. I would end up having to go through the process again, something I did not want to take the time to do.

Frustrated, I asked to roll my own prints on a new card, to which the person doing the fingerprinting retorted under his breath, "You and that Victor guy..." I had to laugh. I knew Victor was a former police officer and I could totally see him saying something about the shoddy job they were doing. I sought him out to tell him what had happened and invited him to join my study group, a small group of mostly non-traditional students who were older and had careers prior to coming to law school.

Victor went through a very long and painful divorce that was finalized during our first year of school. The emotional turmoil caused him to have trouble concentrating and he was placed on academic probation as a result. When he confided this in our study group, we did everything we could to make sure Victor pulled his grades up enough to stay in school.

Now that I was a complete basket case, Victor was my rock. He helped me find a safe, affordable apartment that would take my two dogs. He found some used furniture that was still in good shape that would work for the time being. He organized a moving crew of other law school friends who owned pickups, and together they moved me out of my house and into my new apartment in the heat of July. He made sure I was not by myself for extended periods of time, knowing how easily it is to fall victim to depression. I had a group of friends at my new apartment almost every day, helping me unpack and making sure I ate something.

Once I was unpacked and settled into my new home, I quit wallowing in self-pity long enough to realize all that Victor had done for me. I was so incredibly thankful and wanted him to know how much I appreciated his friendship through all of my turmoil. I didn't have a lot of money to buy him a gift so I offered to make him dinner, knowing he was basically existing on Hamburger Helper® and cans of tuna.

I had kept my emotions between me and God, especially the painful ones, for many years. I rarely opened up to anyone, afraid of being ridiculed or hurt by making myself so vulnerable. For some reason, I didn't have that concern with Victor. We talked for hours that night and when he left I realized that he really understood me. I was grateful to have such a friend and thanked God for putting him in my life.

Victor became one of my best friends in a short amount of time. I could totally be myself with him. He knew the good, the bad, and the ugly. I held nothing back. I wasn't ready to even think about dating anyone again, so I felt safe with him because I knew he wasn't looking for a relationship either. We had both determined we were never getting involved with anyone and definitely never getting married again.

Never say never! We were married at sunrise on August 4, 2006, on Sandy Beach in Oahu, Hawaii. Mike Martindale, pastor of our local church, The Heights Fellowship, officiated. Rachel, my birthmother, and Melanie, my half-sister, stood nearby as witnesses. It was a deeply spiritual ceremony, surrounded by God's amazing handiwork – the colors of the sun rising over the ocean as waves crashed against the shoreline. I had no reservations this time as I committed to spend the rest of my life with my very best friend.

Part III: Beauty for Ashes

The Spirit of the Sovereign Lord is upon me,
for the Lord has anointed me
to bring good news to the poor.
He has sent me to comfort the brokenhearted
and to proclaim that captives will be released
and prisoners will be freed.
He has sent me to tell those who mourn
that the time of the Lord's favor has come,
and with it, the day of God's anger against their enemies.
To all who mourn in Israel,
*he will give a crown of **beauty for ashes**,*
a joyous blessing instead of mourning,
festive praise instead of despair.
In their righteousness, they will be like great oaks
that the Lord has planted for his glory.

Instead of shame and dishonor,
you will enjoy a double share of honor.
You will possess a double portion of prosperity in your land,
and everlasting joy will be yours.
(Isaiah 61:1-3, 7).

Chapter 5: *The Cradle or the Cross: Putting First Things First*

What is the most important thing in your life right now? The one thing you cannot be happy without which occupies your thoughts throughout the day and keeps you staring at the ceiling at night. The one thing that you would sell all you had for and would even beg, borrow and steal in order to get. What is the last thing you think about as you are drifting off to sleep and the first thing you think about when you wake up? Is it God...or is it the overwhelming desire to have a baby? If you are brave enough to get really honest with yourself, you may be surprised at the answer.

Abraham had waited decades for the birth of his son, Isaac. The long waiting period had drawn him closer to God. The Bible doesn't say, but I wonder if Abraham's relationship with God grew more distant after the birth of Isaac. The long-awaited promise was finally here. As much as Abraham loved God, it is so easy to focus more on the gift than the Giver. Isaac may have become a little *too* important to Abraham - possibly more important than God.

> *"Some time later, God tested Abraham's faith. 'Abraham!' God called. 'Yes,' he replied. 'Here I am.' 'Take your son, your only son – yes, Isaac, whom you love so much – and go to the land of Moriah. Go and sacrifice him as a burnt offering on one of the mountains, which I will show you.'*
>
> *The next morning Abraham got up early. He saddled his donkey and took two of his servants with him, along with his son, Isaac. Then he chopped wood for a fire for a burnt offering and set out for the place God had told*

him about. On the third day of their journey, Abraham looked up and saw the place in the distance. 'Stay here with the donkey,' Abraham told his servants. 'The boy and I will travel a little farther. We will worship there, and then we will come right back.'

So Abraham placed the wood for the burnt offering on Isaac's shoulders, while he himself carried the fire and the knife. As the two of them walked on together, Isaac turned to Abraham and said, 'Father?'

'Yes, my son?' Abraham replied.

'We have the fire and the wood,' the boy said, 'but where is the sheep for the burnt offering?'

'God will provide a sheep for the burnt offering, my son,' Abraham answered. And they both walked on together.

When they arrived at the place where God had told him to go, Abraham built an altar and arranged the wood on it. Then he tied his son, Isaac, and laid him n the altar on top of the wood. And Abraham picked up the knife to kill his son as a sacrifice. At that moment the angel of the Lord called to him from heaven, 'Abraham! Abraham!'

'Yes,' Abraham replied. 'Here I am!'

'Don't lay a hand on the boy!' the angel said. 'Do not hurt him in any way, for now I know that you truly fear God. You have not withheld from me even your son, your only son' (Genesis 22:1-12).

This story was absolutely terrifying to me as a child. I remember learning about it in Sunday school on the old flannel boards. The image of young Isaac lying on an altar with his hands and feet tied together was an impression not quickly forgotten. I walked away, wide-eyed and shell shocked, wondering if God would ever tell *my* dad to tie me up and offer me as a sacrifice. And what if it wasn't a test? If nothing else, it was definitely motivation to stay in God's good graces...and my dad's!

I don't believe God ever intended to have Abraham take the life of his only son. I think He wanted to know that Abraham was willing to surrender everything – even Isaac – to the lordship of his Heavenly Father. It was only when Abraham demonstrated that degree of willingness to put the will of God above all else that God was free to pour out His blessings in Abraham's life.

> *Because you have obeyed me and have not withheld even your son, your only son, I swear by my own name that I will certainly bless you. I will multiply your descendants beyond number, like the stars in the sky and the sand on the seashore. And through your descendants all the nations of the earth will be blessed – all because you have obeyed me* (Genesis 22:16-18).

Remember our friend Hannah? Hannah wanted a baby more than life itself. In the midst of great sorrow, she found the strength to cry out to the only One who heard the sound of her heart breaking, the only One who knew just what to say to breathe healing into her soul, the only One who could change her circumstances. She cried to the Lord out of her brokenness and misery, begged Him to give her a son and, in return, promised to give him back to the Lord (I Samuel 1:11).

When Hannah asked God to grant her heart's desire and trusted Him to answer her, something amazing happened. The burden that had been weighing her down all these years was suddenly lifted. It was no longer hers to carry. *She...began to eat again, and she was no longer sad* (I Samuel 1:18).

Like Abraham and Hannah, until we are ready to voluntarily lay down our deepest desires on the altar, God cannot move in our lives the way He wants to. It is so easy to let our own wants and desires overshadow God's plans for us. I wasted many years convincing myself that I knew what was best for me and the best way to go about it. I like to be in control, so it was unnerving to totally and completely relinquish *all* control to God. There were *some* things I was comfortable having Him control, but there were others that I really wanted to keep for myself.

Victor and I had discussed our expectations regarding children at length prior to getting engaged. Though it had been almost four years since my last miscarriage, I was not ready or willing to commit to the idea of getting pregnant again. Victor was fine with that since he had been told by the military that he would not be able to father children anyway. Since we were both in our thirties and about to obtain law degrees, the plan was to focus on our careers, travel, get out of debt as quickly as possible, and just enjoy being married. We agreed to revisit the issue in a year or so to see if we felt differently.

Two months after the wedding I got a call from my doctor's office informing me that my last pap smear had revealed some cellular changes which were cause for concern. I was immediately scheduled to have a biopsy on my cervix. I didn't think that much about it, confident that the biopsy would show everything was fine. It wasn't. I was then scheduled for another procedure to remove a mass of pre-cancerous cells from my cervix. The bad cells ran deeper than the doctors initially thought. My cervix sustained so much damage that my chances of being able to conceive and actually carry a baby to full-term were minimal.

Part of me was devastated by the news. I wasn't ready to have a child in that particular phase of my life, but I still wanted to have that option in the future. Though I knew from experience that genetics have nothing to do with good parenting, I had always pictured my own children to know exactly where they came from and what their biological heritage was. I secretly longed to look into their eyes and see a familiar reflection – that of me or my husband.

I was afraid that if I laid my desire to have a baby on the altar, God would decide that the best way I could serve Him would be to remain childless the rest of my life. I genuinely feared that if I made Him first I would forever be the baby shower hostess but never the mommy-to-be. It sounds crazy, but that is truly how I felt.

Thankfully, God knew that if he gave me what I wanted *when* I wanted it, His purpose for my life would go unfulfilled. God had to show me that even in times and areas where I felt like I was in control, I never was. It was all an illusion, a mirage. He had been in control *the whole time* – not me. It was terrifying, yet freeing at the same time. If God was in control, then I could finally relax and let Him do what He needed to do.

Reflecting back on this "changing of the guard" in my own life, God showed me five Biblical principles that I needed to grab hold of in order to receive spiritual healing from my inability to have children. I needed to know His word and implement it in a very personal way - not just in my head but in my *heart* - in order to walk in victory and be open to the plan

God had for my life. These principles are by no means a magical formula toward getting your prayers answered, nor are they exclusive. They are merely a starting place for you to receive the healing you need in your own life.

Following the discussion on each principle are verses to meditate on or memorize. I urge you not to skim over this part. *Thy word is a lamp unto my feet and a light unto my path* (Psalm 119:105, KJV). It shines light into the darkest corners of our hearts, soothing and healing the things we're afraid to face on our own. It strengthens and encourages us when doubt starts to creep in. Most importantly, it renews our mind with the truth, giving us ammunition against the enemy's lies.

Principle One: Know That God Loves You and Wants Good Things for You

I hesitated to give God control of my desire to have a baby because I did not understand the depth of His love. I had always perceived God's love for me as an obligation. He *loved* me because He *had* to. I wasn't entirely convinced that He actually *liked* me. After all, I was a mess. I made a lot of mistakes and could never seem to get it all together, no matter how good my intentions were. I could never truly be worthy of God's approval.

It took me a long time to realize that God loves me just because I'm His daughter. I don't have to do everything right all the time. He doesn't turn away in shame or disappointment when I fail. He does not want me to live a miserable existence here on earth. He wants me to have a rich and satisfying life (John 10:10). He takes delight in me – just the way that I am (Isaiah 62:4). He rejoices over me with singing (Zephaniah

3:17). I am the apple of His eye (Psalm 17:8). He wants good things for me, infinitely more than I could ever ask or think (Ephesians 3:20).

Once I grasped these truths, meditating on them until they really sunk into the deepest parts of my soul, relinquishing control to my loving Father God was easy. I knew, not just in theory, that He had my best interest at heart. He knew how badly I wanted to be a mom, and He would not withhold any good thing from me as long as I walked with Him in complete submission and obedience (Psalm 84:11). He promised to show me which path to take if I would just seek His will rather than my own (Proverbs 3:6). He wanted to grant my heart's desires and wanted my plans to succeed (Psalm 20:4). All He asked was that I seek Him *above all else* – even above my desire to have a baby – and *then* He would give me everything I needed (Matthew 6:33).

Prescription For Peace

Then Christ will make his home in your hearts as you trust in him. Your roots will grow down into God's love and keep you strong. And may you have the power to understand, as all God's people should, how wide, how long, how high, and how deep his love is (Ephesians 3:17-18).

For as high as the heavens are above the earth, so great is his love for those who fear him (Psalm 103:11, NIV).

I took you from the ends of the earth, from its farthest corners I called you. I said, 'You are my servant;' I have chosen you and have not rejected you. So do not fear, for I am with you; do not be dismayed, for I am your God. I will strengthen you and help you; I will uphold you with my righteous right hand (Isaiah 41:9-10, NIV).

Your love for me is very great. You have rescued me from the depths of death (Psalm 86:13).

"For I know the plans I have for you," declares the Lord, "plans to prosper you and not to harm you, plans to give you hope and a future. Then you will call upon me and come and pray to me, and I will listen to you. You will seek me and find me when you seek me with all your heart" (Jeremiah 29:11-13, NIV).

I have loved you even as the Father has loved me. Remain in my love. When you obey my commandments, you remain in my love, just as I obey my Father's commandments and remain in his love. I have told you these things so that you will be filled with my joy. Yes, your joy will overflow! This is my commandment: Love each other in the same way I have loved you. There is no greater love than to lay down one's life for one's friends (John 15:9-13).

Principle Two: Make God Your Number One Desire

If you have been in church for any amount of time, you know the "Sunday school" hierarchy of priorities: God first, spouse, children, and *then* everything else. But does God *really* have first place in your heart or have you unintentionally stuffed Him in the "everything else" category? God is not satisfied with anything less than first place in our hearts. He's pretty clear about that throughout the Bible, starting with the first commandment: *You must not have any other god but me. For I, the Lord your God, am a jealous God who will not tolerate your affection for any other gods* (Exodus 20:3, 5).

You don't have to have a Buddha statue on your mantle for this to apply to you. Anything can become a 'god' if we rely upon it to determine our value, identity, and reason for living. It might be money, work, recreation, hobbies, food, or a relationship. It could also be the burning desire to have a baby. None of these things are wrong in and of themselves, but if you devote more time and energy thinking about and pursuing them than you do pursuing God, you may have just identified your "god of choice."

If you want to start seeing some breakthroughs in your prayer life, put God back in his rightful place on the throne of your heart. Think about your prayer life for a minute. Do you ask for *His* will or *yours*? Are your prayers limited to variations of "Why aren't you giving me what I want? Don't you love me? Don't you care?"

Think about this: if your spouse spent as much time with you as you are currently spending with God, would you be satisfied with the relationship? What if your spouse only talked to you either to demand something from you (even if it was done politely with all the right flowery words) or to complain that you weren't moving fast enough? Would you feel loved and cherished as a top priority in his life or as significant as the faceless voice behind the drive-thru menu board at Starbucks?

Like me, I'm sure that you long to be the love of your spouse's life. I don't want to be Victor's cook, gardener, maid, nanny, or launderer; rather, the person he shares life with. The first person he calls when something good happens. The first person he confides in when he is scared or unsure of himself. The one he leans on when times are tough. The first one he sees in the morning and the last face he sees before he goes to sleep at night. I want to be his best friend.

That's exactly the kind of relationship that God desires from you. He lovingly pursues you and longs to draw you close to Him. He knows that you will only experience true joy and satisfaction when He is truly first in your life and not just some religious thing you say to impress other people or make yourself feel better. If He is not your first love while you are waiting for your prayers to be answered, He knows He will not be your first love if He gives you what you want.

> *You have persevered and have endured hardships for my name, and have not grown weary. Yet I hold this against you: You have forsaken your first love. Remember the height from which you have fallen! Repent and do the things you did at first. If you do not repent, I will*

come to you and remove your lampstand from its place (Revelation 2:3-5, NIV).

This passage was written to the church in Ephesus both as encouragement and as a warning. God is saying, "Look, you are doing so many things *right* but your heart is not in the right place! Our relationship could be *so much more* than going through the motions. Remember when you first fell in love with me? You loved me so deeply, passionately, enthusiastically! You sought me in everything. *I* was all you ever needed. I was *enough.* Let's get back to that place. Make *me* the main event in your heart again. Make me your best *friend.* I want to bless you with good things. I want to delight in giving you the desire of your heart, but if this desire continues to outweigh your love and desire for me, you cannot fulfill the purpose I have designed you for. I cannot - *will* not - allow that to happen. Even if it means withholding the one thing you want the most."

You probably would not even hesitate to say 'yes' if someone asked if you loved God. You may even be offended by the question. But are you *in love* with Him? Are you actively pursuing an intimate relationship with Him? *[Y]ou must love the Lord your God with* all *your heart,* all *your soul, and* all *your strength* (Deuteronomy 6:5, emphasis added). He doesn't just want what's left after everyone else has taken a piece of you. He wants all of *you* to settle for nothing less than all of *Him.* He wants you to know with absolute certainty that the emptiness you so desperately want to fill with a baby can be only truly filled with Him. *But seek first his kingdom and his righteousness, and all these things will be given to you as well* (Matthew 6:33, NIV).

If it has been a while since you have spent some quality time with God, I encourage you to go no further on our journey together until you have had that opportunity. Get alone with your Father and make it all about *Him* this time rather than all about *you*. Begin with praise and worship. If you're not sure how to do that, turn to the Psalms and read one out loud to Him or play some praise music and just focus on worshipping God for who He *is* rather than what He can do for you. Stand amazed in His presence. The Almighty God of all creation loves you enough to call you His own (I John 3:1).

Thank Him for everything He has blessed you with. Write down each blessing in a prayer journal. Most of us could fill up at least one notebook page, even if it is just things we take for granted such as running water, electricity, food, shelter, a job, or family. Draw a line at the end of your list. If you never received another answer to prayer, never received another blessing, could you be content with what God has already given you?

In her teaching series "Living With Contentment," Joyce Meyer defined contentment as "satisfied to the point where you are no longer disturbed by where you are *now*." So many of us, myself included, think we will be content *when* or content *if* some condition is met rather than being content in the here and now. But it doesn't work that way. Our flesh is never satisfied.

I remember thinking *if I could just find a Christian man to share my life with and get remarried, then I would be happy.* God brought me Victor. We got married. All was well with the world for a while. Then my flesh started screaming again. *I'm tired of school. It's so stressful and time consuming. If we could just graduate from law school and get on with our life, I would be happy.* By the grace of God, we graduated. I was relieved for all of...two months. *If we could just get out of this cramped apartment and into a house, I would be happy.* God hand selected a beautiful house for us. *Now* I should be content, but I really needed a job so I could start paying for that law degree. God provided me with a job. All our needs were met. So I should *really* be content, right? I had an amazing husband, a house in a good neighborhood, an advanced degree, a good job, not to mention great friends and an incredible church home but I was back at it. *If I could just have a baby, then I'll be happy.* How crazy is *that*?

You see where this is going. You probably have your own version of this story. We *all* do. *Just as Death and Destruction are never satisfied, so human desire is never satisfied* (Proverbs 27:20). Contentment is not something that comes to us naturally. It is a *learned* behavior. Paul said, "I have *learned* to be content with whatever I have. I know how to live on almost nothing or with everything. I have *learned* the secret of living in every situation whether it is with a full stomach or empty, with plenty or little. For I can do everything through Christ, who gives me strength" (Philippians 4:11-13, emphasis added).

When all your dreams and expectations seem to be shattering around you, realize that God is all you ever really had and all you really need. Everything else is just a surplus of undeserved blessings. If you cannot be content in Him and content with the blessings He has already given you, why should He give you anything else?

When we let any person, thing, or desire come before God, it throws His perfect order for our lives out of balance. Think of our priorities as a pyramid. When we put God first, we have a firm foundation. Even if everything else were stripped away, we would still have Him as our base, our solid ground on which to rebuild. If we then build our marriage on top of this solid foundation and make it second only to God, it is well supported and able to withstand winds of change and the storms of life because it is supported by the immovable, unchanging solid rock. When we have a strong foundation and a strong marriage, we are then able to be good, godly parents to our children and develop healthy relationships with them. Once our priorities are established, everything else will either line up with them or lose importance.

When we *don't* put God first, it throws all of our other priorities out of balance. Think about that same pyramid we just discussed, but this time it's turned upside down. Now, instead of a solid foundation, you have the pointy tip to build upon. It doesn't work! It's like trying to get one of those spinning tops we used to play with when we were kids to stand perfectly straight. It's not engineered that way. Each and every time you try to ignore its design (and gravity), it will topple over.

The same principle applies to us. When we ignore God's design by failing to seek Him above all else, everything else suffers. Our marriages are no longer stable. Our relationships are rocky. Our moods shift like a swinging pendulum from one extreme to the other. We feel emotionally exhausted and spiritually dead and then we wonder why we feel like everything could easily come crashing down at any minute.

So how do we turn this mess we have made around and get everything back where it is supposed to be? *Seek the kingdom of God above all else, and live righteously, and he will give you everything you need* (Matthew 6:33). Start by *actively pursuing* God above every other thing in your life. You have to be proactive about it because this is not something that comes naturally. It will not happen if you wait to *feel* like it and you cannot wish it into being. Like everything else in life that is of any worth, the active pursuit of God takes discipline and determination. You have to do it *on purpose*. You cannot have the kind of relationship with God that you want and deserve without putting time and effort into it.

We give the first fruits of our income, or the first 10 percent, as a tithe. Why not apply the same principle to your time by giving God the first part of your day? I can already hear the protests: "Well, I'm just not a morning person." Yeah, well, neither am I. I'm not even going to lie about it – I am just *not* a nice person until I have had at least one cup of coffee and quiet time with the Lord. Caffeine and Jesus do wonders for my spirit and allow me to have a much better outlook on my day!

What I have found is that if I make the sacrifice by getting up an hour earlier than I normally do and get alone with God by spending time in His word and talking to Him before I do anything else, I can often hear Him speaking back to me. Not audibly, though He knows I have often wished and prayed for that, but through His word and in my spirit. If I wait until later in the day or at night, my mind is racing with everything that happened that day and it is no longer quiet in my home or in my spirit. I'm not saying that He only speaks in the morning but at least for me, it is the only time He has my full, undivided attention and I can actually hear Him. He's not competing with the noise and distractions. And when I honor Him with the first fruits of my time, He not only multiplies my time but gives me the strength and energy I need to get through the rest of my day.

Another way you can actively pursue God is to practice making Him a part of every aspect of your life. Include Him in every thought, every decision, and every daily menial task of your life. He is with you all the time *anyway*, whether you choose to acknowledge Him or not. You might as well draw upon His tender mercy, strength, wisdom, guidance, grace, and love as much and as often as you can. *I can never escape from your Spirit! I can never get away from your presence!* (Psalm 139:7).

God doesn't live in your church building. It is easy to think of going to church on Sunday mornings as going to "visit" God before coming home to our "real life," where we basically ignore Him the rest of the week. God wants you to talk to Him anywhere, anytime – especially when your heart is breaking.

Set aside any preconceived ideas that you have about prayer. Prayer is simply a conversation with God. There is no reason to make it more complicated than that. You don't have to be alone in a quiet place or in a particular posture. You don't have to use *King James* language unless that's how you talk to your other friends. Start by being open and honest with God about your feelings. If you're mad about what you're going through, tell Him. If you're jealous of the lady in your Sunday school class who just announced she is pregnant with her third baby while you're still waiting for your first one, tell Him. If you don't understand why you going through this agonizing pain and you're angry with God for allowing it, tell Him. He *already knows,* so there's no point in hiding behind what we think He wants to hear or saying what we "should be" feeling in our prayers.

We can hide our true selves, our innermost thoughts and feelings, from a lot of people, even those closest to us, but we cannot hide from God. David wrote, "O Lord, you have examined my heart and know everything about me. You know when I sit down and stand up. You know my thoughts even when I'm far away. You see me when I travel and when I rest at home. You know what I am going to say even before I say it, Lord" (Psalm 139:1-4).

The most intimate relationships are authentic, transparent and honest. Don't worry if you're not where you need to be or if your attitude is not where it needs to be. Invest time in your relationship with God, be honest with Him and He will begin to heal your heart. Your feelings will catch up.

Prescription For Peace

[Y]ou must love the Lord your God with all your heart, all your soul, and all your strength (Deuteronomy 6:5).

Then I realized that my heart was bitter,
and I was all torn up inside.
I was so foolish and ignorant –
I must have seemed like a senseless animal to you.
Yet I still belong to you;
you hold my right hand.
You guide me with your counsel,
leading me to a glorious destiny.
Whom have I in heaven but you?
I desire you more than anything on earth.
My health may fail, and my spirit may grow weak,
but God remains the strength of my heart;
he is mine forever (Psalm 73:21-26, emphasis added).

Seek the Kingdom of God above all else, and live righteously, and he will give you everything you need (Matthew 6:33).

Remain in me, and I will remain in you. For a branch cannot produce fruit if it is severed from the vine, and you cannot be fruitful unless you remain in me. Yes, I am the vine; you are the branches. Those who remain in me, and I in them, will produce much fruit. For apart from me you can do nothing (John 15:4-5).

Dear children, keep away from anything that might take God's place in your hearts (I John 5:21).

Then I pray to you, O Lord. I say, "You are my place of refuge. You are all I really want in life (Psalm 142:5).

Principle Three: Stop Asking Why and Start Trusting

O Lord, how long will you forget me? Forever?
How long will you look the other way?
How long must I struggle with anguish in my soul,
with sorrow in my heart every day?
***But I will trust** in your unfailing love.*
I will rejoice because you have rescued me.
I will sing to the Lord
because he is good to me
(Psalm 13:1-2, 5-6, emphasis added).

One of the biggest obstacles to spiritual healing occurs when we get stuck on trying to figure out "why." *Why me? Why does* she *get to have a baby and* I *don't? Why did God let me get my hopes built up if He knew this was going to happen to me? If God can prevent anything from happening, why did he allow this? Why, God?*

When my nephew was about four years old and I was twelve, we were bunked up together on Christmas Eve. He was just entering the "why" stage and was very concerned because there was a fire burning in the fireplace, preventing Santa from coming down to deliver presents. Desperate for some sleep, I assured him that Santa would be just fine.

"Why?"

"Because Santa wears a fireproof suit."

"Why?"

"Because Mrs. Claus made it that way for him."

"Why?"

"Because a lot of families will have their fireplaces on."

"Why?"

"Because it's cold outside."

"Why?"

"Because it's winter."

"Why?"

This went on and on until I got really frustrated and snapped, "Because I said so!" A tiny voice broke the short period of silence with, "Why?"

I thought a lot about that endless dialogue when I had my own set of questions for God, knowing that each answer to a "why" would only lead to another question. It is normal to have these questions and it is alright to ask them. But in order to experience true healing, we will eventually have to accept that God does not always give straight answers. Some things are just not going to make any sense in our limited human understanding. We have to trade our questions for trust.

I had to do just that when God was beginning to unfold His plan for my life. Victor and I were about to graduate from law school and looking for jobs (since the government actually expected us to pay back all that student loan money). We were both being sought after by the District Attorney's Office in Phoenix, Arizona. Both of us had previous experience in criminal justice. Prior to law school, I had been a probation officer and Vic had been a police officer. Prosecuting was what we went to law school to do. On top of a very competitive salary and amazing benefits, our student loans would be paid by the county after we had worked there for five years. It was a no-brainer on paper. There was no reason to even think twice about it, but something kept nagging at my spirit that it wasn't the right thing to do. The nagging kept me up at night and made me lose my appetite.

One afternoon I was praying about it and asking God about the unsettling feeling that I had about what seemed like a clear answer to our prayers for a good job. All of a sudden I felt God tell me to turn our direction to Amarillo.

I knew it had to be God. Nothing in me wanted to go home. I had clerked there for two summers in a row and it was just different going back after being gone for so long. It was awkward running into people who had known Nathan and me as a couple and having to explain that we were divorced now. A large portion of Nathan's family lived there and I knew eventually I would have to run into one of them. I had no idea how they would react to me or vice versa. There were too many memories there. I had been given a clean slate with Victor and I wanted to go somewhere where both of us would have a fresh start and establish ourselves as a couple.

I convinced myself that I had not heard God correctly. It made absolutely no sense to turn down this amazing offer. Yet day after day I sensed a very strong impression that we needed to be in Amarillo. As much as I tried to shrug it off and as hard as I tried to fight it, it simply would not go away. I continued to lose both weight and sleep until my body and sanity could not take it anymore. Victor and I had booked flights to Phoenix to meet with our superiors, sign paperwork and look for housing. The trip was two weeks away and I knew they would need a commitment from us by then.

I was dreading Victor's reaction when I told him I thought we should cancel our flights and tell them that we weren't coming. We had already talked at great length about what a great blessing the jobs would be. I thought he would laugh at me when I told him I believed God was leading us to Amarillo. He had moved to Fort Worth from New York City and was going crazy in the small town of Lubbock with nothing to do. Amarillo would not be any better. I prayed that God would prepare his heart and help me not to sound like a complete idiot.

I love that we have a God who answers prayer when we have so little faith! Victor listened very intently as I unloaded everything God had been dealing with me about. To my complete surprise, he did not feel the need to slap some sense into me; rather, Victor agreed that if God said that we were supposed to be in Amarillo then that's where we needed to go. We did not need to question Him. We just needed to be obedient.

Victor canceled our flights to Phoenix and we politely declined the amazing opportunities we had been offered. I remember praying, "God, I know you know what you're doing. Teach me to rely on you and forgive my lack of faith. Your plans are so much greater than ours."

I made a few phone calls to some friends in Amarillo who were attorneys to see if there were any jobs available. I also contacted the Potter County Attorney's Office, where I had clerked the summer before. The Criminal Division Chief was very excited that we were considering coming to Amarillo and I had an offer within an hour. It was a decent salary with county benefits, which would be nice since I already had five years invested in the county's retirement system from my years as a probation officer. I felt certain that this is where I needed to be.

The other opportunity was to go into private practice at a friend's law firm. Victor and I were offered one year of rent-free office space until we could establish ourselves in the community and get on our feet. We could keep all of the income we brought in. After the first year, we would work something out as far as either rent or contributing a percentage of our income to the firm. There were no benefits – no health or life insurance and no retirement. We were given ballpark figures on what to expect for average income – some months we could earn a six-figure income. Other months, we may earn nothing at all. The whole "you eat what you kill" concept blew my mind. I didn't think I could live like that. How would we budget?

I walked away from the meeting feeling even more certain that I needed to be at the County Attorney's Office for my own peace of mind if nothing else. Victor liked the idea of being in private practice and was up for the challenge. He took our friend's offer right away.

I was about to call the Criminal Division Chief to accept the offer when I got that same nudging in my spirit again. *What now, God?* All of a sudden my peace about going to the county went completely out the window. I was scared to death. I felt the Lord was telling me to go into private practice with Vic.

"WHAT?!? Are you *kidding* me? With no benefits? No set salary? At least *one* of us needs those things or we are going to drown!"

I was in full blown hysteria when God calmly told me that the only thing we truly needed was Him. He would take care of me, just as He always had. The words of Jeremiah 29:11 came to mind – *For I know the plans I have for you...plans to prosper you and not to harm you, plans to give you a hope and a future.*

I knew without a doubt that even though it made no sense, I needed to go into private practice with Victor.

Those first few months of private practice were some of the scariest times in my life. The instability was nerve wrecking in so many ways, yet I would not change that period in our lives for anything. We were totally and completely reliant on God to take care of us. He never let us down. Not once. He provided for us in ways that far exceeded anything we could have ever imagined. More importantly, He had put me in private practice for a very specific purpose.

Our lives started taking a new direction on Thanksgiving of 2007. For some reason, I had been thinking a lot about starting a family of our own. The timing was horrible. We were drowning in student loans and personal debt, our income was totally "feast or famine," and we had no insurance. On top of that, I knew my chances of getting and staying pregnant were slim to none and I knew it would probably be a long time before we could afford an adoption, but I just could not get the thought of having a baby out of my mind.

On Thanksgiving night, after playfully breaking the wishbone with Victor, I rested my head on his chest as he held me close and asked what I had wished for. Feeling fairly confident that he would either laugh or freak out, I spoke barely above a whisper when I said, "a baby".

There was a long silence and I held my breath as I prepared myself for a speech about how it just wasn't the right time. I was completely shocked that Vic was actually open to discussing it. We decided to try to get pregnant for a year, knowing we would probably be unsuccessful, and then start seriously looking into adoption. We knew that God's timing was perfect and we would trust Him to know when the right time was. We had complete faith, though as small as a mustard seed at times, that He would bless us some way, somehow.

"Lord," I prayed, "If you can heal our bodies and allow us to have a child of our own - that would be awesome. If not, lead us to the right agency or pair us with the right birthmother."

I *thought* I was praying the right prayer with the right heart. That's what I get for thinking. God used this opportunity to teach me something very crucial. I had just finished my prayer when I heard Him speak to my spirit.

"You really don't know me, do you?"

"What do you *mean* I don't know you? I've known you all my life, Lord."

"If you knew me, really *knew* me, you would believe me. You would know that there is nothing too big for me."

I was dumbfounded. I had believed in God all my life and I believed the Bible was true, but there was a part of me deep down inside that didn't believe He could really help me - that some things were too much to ask of Him. I kept my prayers small and my faith even smaller.

I was immediately reminded of the father who had brought his afflicted son to Jesus. The father had been dealing with the ugliness of his son's condition so long that he honestly could not imagine what it would be like to have his son completely restored. "If you can do anything, take pity on us and help us" (Mark 9:22, NIV). *If.* The very same word I had used. *If* you can heal our bodies. As the scriptures slowly began to sink in, I felt Jesus speaking directly to me. *"If you can?" said Jesus. "Everything is possible for him who believes"* (Mark 9:23, NIV).

I believed in my *head* but I did not believe in my *heart*. Jesus had conquered death itself yet a small part of me did not believe He could help me. Or maybe it wasn't so much that I thought He *couldn't* but that He *wouldn't*. I remembered asking for Mary Ann's complete healing and believing He would do it. When He didn't, I was devastated. I had not trusted Him with the innermost depths of my heart ever since. I could ask Him for small, day-to-day things but I did not trust Him with the big things, things that meant the most to me.

My distrust and unbelief had become a stronghold, blocking the power of God in my life. I remembered reading a verse in Matthew during my quiet time that both challenged and frightened me: *According to your faith will it be done to you* (Matthew 9:29, NIV). Big faith, big answers. Little faith, little answers. *Oh, Father God. Help me overcome my unbelief.*

Once the enemy realized his stronghold had been revealed and that I was actively praying God's word against it, he immediately put stumbling blocks in my path to try to steal my hope, peace and joy. While I was busy trying to plant God's promises in my heart, Satan was trying to uproot them.

A family member called to say she had just found out she was pregnant. She was unmarried and the father was long gone. She had never held a steady job, partly due to severe emotional problems, and often had to depend on other family members to bail her out financially.

I got off the phone and cried. *Why? I mean* really. She had absolutely nothing to offer a baby. It was not only unfair, but seemed *cruel* that God would entrust *her* with a precious baby when I didn't think she deserved one.

The doctor's words played over and over in my head - our chances of having a baby were minimal at best. Despair and hopelessness set in as I replayed those conversations again and again in my mind, like constantly hitting rewind and play on an old cassette tape recorder.

My faith seemed to wax and wane like the ocean tide, though I longed to be steadfast. A still small voice would interrupt my thoughts and gently ask, *"Do you trust me? Do you believe in me?"* God showed me that my faith could not be based on my feelings. I had to learn to set them aside. Feelings are fickle but God's word is the same yesterday, today and forever (Hebrews 13:8). *What I feel isn't real.* I *feel* forgotten but God says He has written me on the palm of His hand (Isaiah 49:16). I *feel* abandoned but God says he will never leave me nor forsake me (Hebrews 13:5). Every time I would feel something that undermined my faith, I would claim God's promise that through Him *all* things are possible (Matt 9:26) and hold tightly to the hope He had given me.

115

Prescription For Peace

My future is in your hands (Psalm 31:15).

Take delight in the Lord,
and he will give you your heart's desires.
Commit everything you do to the Lord.
Trust him, and he will help you (Psalm 37:4-5).

You are the God who performs miracles (Psalm 77:14, NIV).

Keep on asking, and you will receive what you ask for. Keep on seeking, and you will find. Keep on knocking, and the door will be opened to you. For everyone who asks, receives. Everyone who seeks, finds. And to everyone who knocks, the door will be opened (Matthew 7:7-8).

You can ask for anything in my name, and I will do it, so that the Son can bring glory to the Father. Yes, ask me for anything in my name, and I will do it (John 14:13-14).

And we know that in all things God works together for good for those who love Him and are called according to His purpose (Romans 8:28, NIV).

Dear brothers and sisters, when troubles come your way, consider it an opportunity for great joy. For you know that when your faith is tested, your endurance has a chance to grow. So let it grow, for when your endurance is fully developed, you will be perfect and complete, needing nothing (James 1:2-4).

You do not have what you want because you don't ask God for it (James 4:2).

And it is impossible to please God without faith. Anyone who wants to come to him must believe that God exists and that he rewards those who sincerely seek him (Hebrews 11:6).

And we will receive from him whatever we ask because we obey him and do the things that please him (1 John 3:22).

Principle Four: Make A Decision to Have Joy

A positive attitude will not solve all the problems in the world, but it will annoy enough people to make it worth the effort.
– Unknown

He that is down need fear no fall. – John Bunyan

Most women are familiar with the famous line from *Jerry Maguire* where Tom Cruise looks at Renee Zellweger and says, "You...complete me."[6] Some of you are tearing up just thinking about it. I mean, what an incredible thing to say to someone, am I right?

Well, have you ever been around someone who does the opposite? Someone who incessantly wallows in her own misery and drains you of every ounce of energy? Someone who makes you want to look at her and say, "You...deplete me." Reality check: are *you* that person?

Everyone loves a good pity party. Especially women. As little girls, we milked each scraped knee or hurt feeling for all it was worth; running to the arms of our mother (or father) who would hold us close, stroke our hair and say, "There, there. Poor baby." As teenagers we counted on our close friends to bring chocolate and tissues as we sat around the stereo, listening to sad love songs and crying over our first heartbreak while they assured us we were too good for him anyway. Most of us still have something in us that longs for that soft place to land when life treats us unfairly.

As a Christ follower, I had always assumed that was part of Jesus' job title. After all, the Bible says to cast our cares on

---

[6] Crowe, Cameron. <u>Jerry Maguire</u>. TriStarPictures, 2002.

him because He cares for us (I Peter 5:7). *He took up our infirmities and carried our sorrows* (Isaiah 53:4, NIV). I pictured Him holding me and rocking me, like my dad did when I was a little girl with a skinned elbow. What I discovered through studying scripture absolutely turned my world upside down.

> *Now there is in Jerusalem near the Sheep Gate a pool, which in Aramaic is called Bethesda and which is surrounded by five covered colonnades. Here a great number of disabled people used to lie – the blind, the lame, the paralyzed. One who was there had been an invalid for* **thirty-eight** *years. When Jesus saw him lying there and learned that he had been in this condition for a long time, he asked him, "Do you want to get well?"*
>
> *"Sir," the invalid replied, "I have no one to help me into the pool when the water is stirred. While I am trying to get in, someone else goes down ahead of me."*
>
> *Then Jesus said to him, "***Get up!*** Pick up your mat and walk." At once the man was cured; he picked up his mat and walked* (John 5:2-9, NIV, emphasis mine).

You may have heard this story so many times that you were tempted to skim over it, but please don't miss what was going on here. The man had been an invalid for *thirty-eight years*. Thirty-eight years! That is a long time to live paralyzed and discouraged, wouldn't you agree?

Jesus certainly thought so. Notice his question to the man. *"Do you want to get well?"* If we were really honest with ourselves, we would admit that sometimes we don't actually want to get well. Like the man by the pool, we have lived with our pain or infirmity so long that it feels like it is a part of us or maybe it gets us the attention and sympathy we feel we deserve. We are scared of what life would be like if it were suddenly gone. Things would not ever be the same. *We* would not ever be the same. Change can be terrifying.

Sometimes we just want to keep wallowing in our misery and make excuses for why we can't seem to snap out of it. I don't know about you, but I kind of feel sorry for the poor guy by the pool – probably because his answer sounds exactly like something I would have said: "They won't help me and *then* they cut in line!" Here he is, throwing himself a royal pity party and inviting Jesus to join in.

We might expect Jesus to kneel down, pat the guy on the shoulder and say, "I'm so sorry that happened to you. Poor thing. Let *me* help you get into the pool." But what does Jesus say? "Get *up!*" And not only *that*, but "Pick up your mat and walk!" In other words, get up and then *do* something with yourself! Quit lying around like a bump on a log, expecting everyone to coddle you!

Consequently, Jesus gave the very same response to the paralytic who was lowered through the ceiling to receive healing: "Get up, take your mat and go home" (Matthew 9:6, NIV). He even gave this command to *dead people*, from a child (Mark 5:38-43) to his close friend, Lazarus (John 11:43). At least, like Peter, *I now realize that how true it is that God does not show favoritism* (Acts 10:34).

Why did Jesus respond so harshly? Was he being insensitive? Mean? Cruel? No, not at all. Jesus was challenging the man to get over his self-pity before it confined him to a lifetime of misery and emptiness. We are totally ineffective as

Christ-followers when we are in that kind of condition. We cannot reach out to others in need because we are so focused on our own needs. We cannot serve because we feel a sense of entitlement to *be* served. We let our joy become dependent on our circumstances and lose our hope when things do not go the way we want them to. What Jesus was trying to say to the man at the pool was simply this: "Enough already! Stop feeling sorry for yourself. Stop looking at what *is* and start focusing on what *can be* if you will put your trust in me. Stop making excuses about how you "can't help" how you feel. Yes, you *can*! *'Do not let your hearts be troubled. Trust in God; trust also in me'"* (John 14:1, NIV, emphasis mine). Do not let yourself automatically default into discouragement every time things do not go the way you want them to. *Don't be dejected and sad, for the joy of the Lord is your strength!* (Nehemiah 8:10). *Choose* to have joy! Get up!

You may feel like you have absolutely nothing to be joyful about. I've been there. Let me tell you from experience that joy will continue to elude you as long as your focus remains on your circumstances and all of the things you do not have. True joy comes from realizing the consistency of God's love and presence in our lives. The tides of life may rise and fall around us but that does not mean our emotions have to follow its course. *"In the world you will have tribulation and trials and distress and frustration; but be of good cheer [take courage; be confident, certain, undaunted]! For I have overcome the world. [I have deprived it of power to harm you and have conquered it for you]"* (John 16:33, Amplified Bible). You are not powerless over your emotions. Jesus has already set you free from their hold on

120

you if you will just draw upon His strength and call upon the power of the Holy Spirit that is already living within you! Joyce Meyer once said that you can either be pitiful or powerful but not both. Which is it going to be?

In his article entitled *Resist Discouragement*, Pastor Rick Warren wrote:

> If you're discouraged, that's your choice. You have chosen to be discouraged. Discouragement is always a choice. It comes from thinking discouraging thoughts – and you can change your thoughts any time. You have a choice of what you're going to focus on: either your purpose or your problems, God's power or your weakness, Christ or your circumstances. It's your choice.[7]

I had grown angry, discouraged, and bitter. I was like the Israelites, groaning in the desert after being delivered from a life of slavery (*see* Exodus 15:22 - 16:36). I was so busy focusing on groaning about everything that I was completely blinded to the abundance of blessings that God had poured into my life.

The scales suddenly fell from my eyes and I saw how ungrateful and ugly I had been. It was as if God had lovingly raised my head with His hand, looked me in the eye and asked, "Why should I give you anything else when you do nothing but complain about what I have already given you?"

It was the most humbling experience I have ever had. I bowed my head, no longer in condemnation but in confession. I was in complete agreement with God. My prayer that day was for Him to purge away everything within me that was not of Him. Every personality quirk, every inherited bend toward negativity,

---

[7] Warren, Rick. *Resist Discouragement.* Called To Be Free. Web. 30 Nov, 2006.

every childhood vow, every bitter root that had unwittingly been planted in my spirit that was choking out the very life Jesus had died for me to have, I asked Him to strip it all away until nothing was left but Jesus.

I spent the next few weeks in "detox" from all of my negative attitudes and thinking patterns. I created play lists of praise and worship songs that spoke to my heart, songs that encouraged me and forced me to get my mind off of myself and onto God. Every time a discouraging thought tried to work its way into my mind or out of my mouth, I replaced it with God's word, taking captive every thought to make it obedient to Christ (2 Corinthians 10:5). I had a choice to make. I could continue to be miserable or I could choose joy.

There is a time to mourn and a time to heal (Ecclesiastes 3:3-4). It's O.K. to mope around for a little while. It's *not* O.K. to lay down our mat and permanently camp out there. The only way to receive healing is to get up! Be thankful! Have joy! So what are you waiting for? Get up, dust yourself off and move forward.

Arise, my darling,
my beautiful one, and come with me.
See! The winter is past,
the rains are over and gone.
Flowers appear on the earth;
the season of singing has come...
Arise, come, my darling;
My beautiful one, come with me
(Song of Songs 2:10-13, NIV).

Prescription For Peace

I will be filled with joy because of you.
I will sing praises to your name, O Most High (Psalm 9:2).

You have turned my mourning into joyful dancing.
You have taken away my clothes of mourning
and clothed me with joy, that I might sing praises to you
and not be silent (Psalm 30:11-12).

I will be glad and rejoice in your unfailing love,
for you have seen my troubles,
and you care about the anguish of my soul (Psalm 31:7).

Sorrow and mourning will disappear,
and they will be filled with joy and gladness (Isaiah 35:10).

Until now you have not asked for anything in my name. Ask
and you will receive, and your joy will be complete
(John 16:24, NIV).

Be joyful always; pray continually; give thanks in all
circumstances, for this is God's will for you in Christ Jesus
(1 Thessalonians 5:16-18, NIV).

So be truly glad. There is wonderful joy ahead, even though you
have to endure many trials for a little while. These trials will
show that your faith is genuine. It is being tested as fire tests
and purifies gold – though your faith is far more precious than
mere gold. So when your faith remains strong through many
trials, it will bring you much praise and glory and honor on the
day when Jesus Christ is revealed to the whole world.
(1 Peter 1:6-7).

Principle Five: Wait With Enthusiastic Expectancy

No one in our society likes to wait. We have grown very accustomed to drive-through convenience. We want our fast food orders to be filled in five minutes or less. If we take the time to go to a "sit down" restaurant, the first thing we want to know is how long we can expect to wait. If we don't want to wait that long, we have no problem going somewhere else. *We* want to decide how long we are going to wait and do not like indefinite waiting periods.

Waiting conjures up images of sitting still in complete boredom until it's our turn. Think about the dynamics of a doctor's office waiting room, especially in those "urgent care" type centers. If you look around, you will see people either glancing at the clock or their watch every so often, folding their arms, taking in deep breaths and letting out loud sighs or tapping their feet. Every time the door of the "inner sanctum" opens, everyone in the waiting room looks up and listens expectantly, hoping it is *their* name that will be called this time. But, *sigh*, only one name will be called and while that person is hurriedly grabbing his things and heading through the door, the rest of the motley crew sink back in their chairs with a slump.

Part of living in contentment involves waiting on God. This is a different kind of waiting. It is *actively* hoping and *expectantly* looking forward to what God is going to do. It is easy to get excited when we see God's hand at work in our life. It is when we do *not* see that it becomes difficult. When the waiting period is longer than we expected or hoped for, we have a tendency to think He must need our help moving things along. The results are always disaster and chaos when we take matters into our own hands rather than waiting on what God has for us.

A prime example of this is the story of Abraham and Sarah. Abraham dealt with discontentment just like we do. In the passage we discussed earlier, Abraham laments, "O Sovereign Lord, what good are all your blessings when I don't even have a son?" God not only promises Abraham a son, but declares that his descendants will be more numerous than the stars (Genesis 15:4-5). He had a direct promise from God even though his wife, Sarah, had struggled with infertility for many, many years.

The Bible doesn't say how much time went by after this promise was made. It may have been months or even years. We don't really know. All we know is that Sarah had given up hope of ever becoming pregnant, promise or no promise. In her impatience, she devises a plan to make it happen on *her* timetable and through her own efforts.

"The Lord has prevented me from having children. Go and sleep with my servant. Perhaps I can have children through her." And Abraham agreed with [this] proposal (Genesis 16:2). Abraham *agreed*...the same Abraham whom God declared as righteous for his faith (Genesis 15:6). If Abraham and Sarah would have just waited on God, they could have saved themselves a lot of heartache.

If you are familiar with the story, you know what happens next. If you're not, you can probably guess. Sarah's servant, Hagar, becomes pregnant by Abraham and begins to openly disrespect Sarah's authority just as Sarah had disrespected God's

(Genesis 16:4-5). What took place over the following months and years is heartbreaking: broken relationships; finger pointing; marital strife; an innocent child, despised and ultimately kicked out of his father's house, never really belonging; bitter tears; sleepless nights full of regret. All of this mess because Sarah didn't want to wait on God. It was thirteen years later before the promised son, Isaac, arrived, but Sarah probably would have waited thirteen more if she could undo all of the damage she set in motion by stepping ahead of God.

If you are still waiting for God to answer your prayer for a child, I want to encourage you once again with the words of Pastor Rick Warren:

> "God's delay is not a denial. Just because you haven't had the answer or the miracle yet, that doesn't mean God isn't going to do it eventually. It simply means not yet! Maturity is knowing the difference between, 'No,' and 'Not yet,' between a delay and a denial. God says, 'Don't become discouraged. Resist discouragement'. Because there are going to be delays in your life...God tests you, not for him to find out what's inside of you but for *you* to find out what's inside of you. He tests you so you'll know your level of commitment, and he tests you so that you can know his faithfulness."[8]

Take heart, dear one. He has not forgotten you.

---

[8] Warren, Rick. *Resist Discouragement*. Called To Be Free. Web. 30 Nov, 2006.

Prescription For Peace

Listen to my voice in the morning, Lord.
Each morning I bring my requests to you and wait expectantly
(Psalm 5:3).

Wait patiently for the Lord.
Be brave and courageous.
Yes, wait patiently for the Lord (Psalm 27:14).

Be still and know that I am God! (Psalm 46:10).

I wait quietly before God,
for my victory comes from him.
He alone is my rock and my salvation,
my fortress where I will never be shaken (Psalm 62:1-2).

He gives the childless woman a family, making her a happy
mother (Psalm 113:9).

So the Lord must wait for you to come to him
so he can show you his love and compassion.
For the Lord is a faithful God.
Blessed are those who wait for his help (Isaiah 30:18).

As for me, I look to the Lord for help.
I wait confidently for God to save me,
And my God will certainly hear me (Micah 7:7).

But they that wait upon the Lord shall renew their strength;
they shall mount up with wings as eagles; they shall run, and
not be weary; and they shall walk, and not faint
(Isaiah 40:31, KJV).

Therefore we do not lose heart. Though outwardly we are
wasting away, yet inwardly we are being renewed day by day.
For our light and momentary troubles are achieving for us an
eternal glory that far outweighs them all. So we fix our eyes not
on what is seen, but on what is unseen
(2 Corinthians 4:16-18, NIV).

Chapter 6: Delayed But Not Forgotten

And the Lord remembered Hannah (I Samuel 1:19, NIV).

With man this is impossible, but with God all things are possible (Matthew 19:26, NIV).

"When one door of happiness closes, another opens; but often we look so long at the closed door that we do not see the one which has been opened for us." – Helen Keller

An unfamiliar car caught my eye as I pulled into the firm parking lot at 7:55 a.m. that December morning. I glanced at the red file sticking up from my briefcase. My secretary had a color coded filing system. Family cases were in red files because family clients are always out for blood. A green label on the tab stood for money, or the lack thereof, since the court was paying my bill.

So who *was* this indigent family client anyway? Name: Lowe, Valerie*. She was early. I was impressed she even showed up. I had spent weeks hunting her down. The phone number she had provided the court had been disconnected and the letters I sent her had been returned "Attempted: Unknown". I closed my eyes and took a deep, cleansing breath as I closed the car door with my elbow, sloshing gourmet coffee on the crisp white sack holding my honey almond bagel with honey almond cream cheese, a treat I allowed myself every Friday as a reward for getting through the week.

I had been a licensed attorney for a grand total of 46 days and was already having serious second thoughts. I went to law school to help people, to make a difference, and to finally earn the respect I felt I deserved. Now that I had experienced a small

128

taste of what being an attorney was really like, I just had to laugh at my naiveté.

I had already established that, at least in family law, the clients don't really want your help, they want revenge. They want whatever is going to cause the least amount of effort or pain on their part while making it as excruciating as possible for the other party. And *respect*? Who was *I* kidding? Lawyers are the butt of a whole slew of jokes and one of the least respected professions. We are perceived as ambulance chasers and money hungry thieves who make big promises and over-bill clients.

Now I was stuck. Tens of thousands of dollars in debt for my education left me with no choice but to suck it up and try to put as much enthusiasm and compassion as I could muster into my new life as "Attorney at Law."

These thoughts were rolling through my mind as I balanced my briefcase, purse, lunch bag, coffee and bagel in one hand while I fumbled with keys and pushed open the creaky back door with my hip, making my way to the musty corner office with the green carpet and the exhilarating view of the Salvation Army across the street.

The completed client questionnaire packet for Ms. Lowe was waiting on my desk. She must have been waiting for a while now. Plopping down in my faux leather chair, I pulled the now coffee-stained file from my briefcase and flipped through her paperwork.

Twenty-three years of age, divorced, three children - one of whom had been removed by Child Protective Services (CPS) eight months ago on the grounds of abuse and neglect. This is why she is here today. Every parent who has had a child removed involuntarily has the right to legal representation.

It appears Ms. Lowe has been cooperating with CPS. She claims she has completed a psychological evaluation and is currently in parenting classes and drug/alcohol outpatient therapy. I made a note to verify these things. As a former probation officer I had already learned that people who are backed into a corner will say and do just about anything to get themselves out of trouble.

Ms. Lowe had been waiting long enough. I took one last sip of coffee to wash down my bagel and stood up to brush crumbs off of my suit before going to get her. Though I did not expect to like Ms. Lowe from reading her file, almost instantly I felt a connection to her. She was a little rough around the edges with an eyebrow piercing and a street-smart attitude, but she was real.

Valerie, as she had insisted I call her, was very open about the situation that got her involved with CPS. She had gotten involved in a relationship with someone who had a drug problem – someone she thought she could change. Instead, as is usually the case, he ended up dragging her down with him. Valerie had been physically and emotionally abused by this man. She had lost everything she had worked so hard for: her own apartment, a good job, a car, a bank account, and now her son. It was exactly the type of wakeup call she needed. Valerie had gotten out of the relationship, moved in with her father, and was working nights so she could comply with all of the CPS requirements during the day. Her whole life now revolved around getting her son back. I really had to marvel at her determination.

There was one other thing, Valerie said. She was pregnant again with this man's child. "Of *course* you are," I thought to myself. I wanted to roll my eyes and sigh out loud, but I refrained. Unplanned baby number four. *Really God?*

To my surprise, Valerie said she knew she could not keep this baby and had already made up her mind to pursue adoption. She asked if I knew anything about the adoption process, as she was worried she would have to come up with money that she didn't have. Planned Parenthood had given her a sheet of paper with a list of adoption agencies on it, but she was overwhelmed and confused by the whole thing.

My heart softened. Valerie was more mature than I had given her credit for. She was thinking about what was best for the baby rather than what would be easiest for her.

I shared my own adoption story, how my parents had raised me to have respect for my birthmother and the difficult decision she had made, and that I have a very good relationship with her now that I'm an adult. Valerie listened intently and her eyes filled with tears every once in a while, prompting her to look away, shake it off, and look back at me.

"That's exactly what I want for this baby. He deserves so much more than I could ever give him. I just don't want him to hate me," she said.

"It's a boy?" I asked.

"Actually, I haven't had my sonogram yet, but I just have a feeling it's a boy."

"He won't hate you, Valerie. Hopefully he will go to the right family and they will explain to him that you loved him so much that you did what was best for him. Not what was best or easiest for *you*, but what was best for *him*."

I was currently serving on the Board of Directors for Special Delivery Infant Adoptions[9] and knew both Cindy Gilliland, the director, and Carissa Wingate, the case manager who worked with birthmothers, very well. I knew they would take good care of Valerie if this is the route she decided to go, so I gave her Carissa's card and told Valerie to give them a call.

I thought about Valerie often over the next few weeks, wondering if she had contacted an agency or if she changed her mind. I prayed for the baby's health and that he would be placed with a family that loved the Lord and would raise him to respect Valerie and view his adoption as a special gift.

Meanwhile, the New Year had just begun and I had psyched myself into believing I was pregnant. I wanted to be so badly and wanted to surprise Victor on his birthday with the news that he would be a daddy. I had only been off of the pill for 3 months and my cycles were still all over the place, but when I didn't start my period when I *thought* I should, I headed to the drug store for a test.

The best time to take one of these things, according to the package, is first thing in the morning, so I reluctantly waited. I barely slept, counting the hours until morning, only to have a blank white space stare back at me when the two agonizing

[9] For more information, go to www.specialdeliveryadoptions.org

minutes had passed. My eyes stung and a lump welled up in my throat, but I forced myself to stop the meltdown before it started.

I took a deep breath and prayed, "Your timing, Lord. Not mine. You know what's best. You are all I need. I will trust you while I wait."

Two weeks later, Valerie and I were leaving a status conference at CPS when she said she needed to talk to me. She had a nervous look mixed with pure determination and it worried me a little.

"There's something I want to ask you." Valerie looked at her shoes and began to fidget a little. "Do you know anything about private adoptions?"

"Yes. Did you find a couple to adopt the baby?"

"Well, maybe. My counselor knows some people in Arizona that are interested, but that's the thing." She took a deep breath. "I don't want this baby to go to someone I don't know, so...do you want him?"

I was sure I had not heard her correctly. I dropped my briefcase and the noise brought me back to my senses. I looked around for a chair, feeling a sudden desperate need to sit down before my knees gave way. It was like Reese Witherspoon's line in *Legally Blonde*, "I'm sorry. I just hallucinated. Now, *what*?"[10]

"Seriously, Clair. You and your husband are both lawyers and I know this baby will be well taken care of."

I wanted to hug her while screaming and jumping up and down, but I refrained. It took me a minute to compose myself and come up with something half-way intelligent to say. I told

[10] Luketic, Robert. <u>Legally Blonde</u>. MGM Studios, 2001.

133

her that I obviously needed to discuss this with Victor, but to please not make a decision until I had a chance to do that.

My hands were trembling as I opened the car door and made the short drive back to the office. So many thoughts flooded my mind. I wanted to allow myself to be excited at the prospect of being a mommy in four short months but the practical side of me knew I shouldn't get my hopes built up. There were so many unknowns, so many unanswered questions. There was mass chaos going on in my head.

I walked into Victor's office and shut the door behind me. He whirled around in his chair, eyes wide.

"What's wrong?" he asked.

"Do you want a baby?" I could feel a sheepish smile working its way across my face.

"Yeah. Do you have one?"

I closed my eyes and took a deep breath. *No, really.*

"Yes, honey. I have one in my purse," I replied, my voice dripping with sarcasm. "Do you want to *adopt* one?"

I explained what had gone on that morning and Vic didn't even hesitate. He was definitely interested and told me to set up a meeting with her so we could ask more questions and make sure this was going to be a right fit for everyone. We needed to know what she expected from us and needed to figure out what we expected from her. I immediately called Valerie and, trying not to sound overly anxious to the point of scaring the poor girl, left a message that Vic and I would like to meet with her to talk about this further.

It was days before Valerie returned my call. I checked messages constantly, paced the floor, and bit the inside corners of my mouth to the consistency of raw hamburger meat until I heard from her. I had said I wouldn't get my hopes built up and wouldn't get attached, but it was too late. The tiny, unborn baby had already taken up residence in my heart.

Valerie agreed to meet at my office on a Friday afternoon. I invited Carissa Wingate from Special Delivery, to facilitate. Still not entirely convinced that Valerie would show, I told Carissa to wait until she heard from me before making the trip downtown.

Victor was meeting with a client upstairs and I was trying hard to keep my mind busy, flipping through a client file and trying to take notes when my secretary burst into my office and announced that Valerie was here. Thank you, Jesus!

I tried to stand up but my knees were complete Jell-O® and I fell back into my swivel chair, scattering loose paperwork all over the floor. My secretary pursed her lips and shook her head sympathetically.

"Why don't I bring Ms. Lowe back in about five minutes?" she kindly suggested.

I was a nervous wreck. The minute Valerie walked in the door, my hands started shaking and my bottom lip kept doing this weird trembling thing as I managed to smile and hand Valerie a scrapbook of our wedding and a copy of a local magazine article I had recently been featured in regarding my own adoption.

"I don't know why I'm so nervous about this. I ask people questions for a living," I said, trying to break the uncomfortable silence.

"Not about this. It's O.K. to be nervous. I know *I* am."

135

Despite her tough exterior, Valerie had a kind heart and a sweet spirit that would come out of hiding every once in a while. I excused myself to call Carissa and let Vic know Valerie was here, while Valerie intently read the magazine article I had given her.

"This is exactly what I want for my baby," she said, pointing to the glossy magazine article with my picture. "Have you thought of names?"

I hope she doesn't hate them, I thought to myself.

"Ryan Cade, if it's a boy, and Brooklyn Faith, if it's a girl." She smiled. "I like those."

As discreetly as I could, I breathed a sigh of relief as Carissa let herself in, offered a warm introduction to Valerie and sat next to her. Carissa talked easily to Valerie as if she had known her for years.

"First of all, I want you to know that although I am a friend of Victor and Clair's, in this situation I am here for *you*. There are a lot of emotions involved in placing a baby for adoption. All of them are perfectly normal. Along the way, there may be questions or feelings that you may be uncomfortable sharing with Victor and Clair. If and when that happens, I want you to know you have someone to call." Carissa jotted down her cell phone number on the back of a card and handed it to Valerie. "It's always on. No matter what time of day or night, call me if you need me."

Victor quietly let himself in and leaned up against the side of the desk.

"So, Valerie, why don't you start by telling us why you want to place this baby for adoption," Carissa gently said.

136

Valerie took a deep breath.

"Well, I'm already a single mom of three. My son, who has special health needs, is in foster care and I am working very hard to get him back. I love my kids more than anything in this world and if I were in a better situation right now..." her voice drifted off and started to quiver. "I just want this baby to have so much more than I can give. I want him...or her...to grow up with two parents who love each other and to have opportunities that I can't offer. There is no way that I can provide for another baby right now."

Valerie wiped away a single tear that was making its way down her cheek.

"Sorry," she whispered quietly, while reaching for a tissue on my desk.

My heart went out to her and I wanted to go to her, put my arms around her and let her cry on my shoulder, but Carissa locked her gaze with mine and gave me a look that said to stay put.

"It's O.K. to cry. I would worry about you if you didn't." Carissa gently put her hand on top of Valerie's before moving on. "Now tell me why you picked Victor and Clair to be this baby's parents."

Valerie gripped her tissue, looked up at me through bloodshot eyes and smiled.

"I don't really know Victor and I barely know Clair. But I can tell they are good people, caring people. My mom is a great judge of character and after she met Clair, she told me, 'that's who needs to be raising this baby'. I think she's right. I like the fact that Clair's adopted so she can identify with the baby. She

137

turned out great. I mean, she's an attorney...and Victor's an attorney so they are smart people with ambition. I want my baby to be like them."

I met Victor's gaze and knew exactly what he was thinking. *This may actually happen.* We could be parents in the next four months.

Carissa must have known what we were thinking, too, because she then turned to us.

"Clair, Vic, why do you want to be this baby's parents?"

Wow. How could I possibly express everything that was on my heart? Victor nodded at me to go first, so I took a deep breath and said a prayer that God would give me the right words to reflect my deepest emotions.

"First of all, Victor and I are not only husband and wife, we are best friends. We do everything together and are involved in every detail of each other's lives. We work together, which some people think is crazy, but we really enjoy it. We are just very close, we love being together, and I wouldn't have it any other way. We have so much love in our home..." my voice began to crack and I had to pause to blink away tears before continuing.

"We have so much love in our home that we want more than anything to share that with a child. We knew before we got married that having a family together may be impossible due to health complications, but we believe in God and have been praying for a miracle.

I thought God would answer our prayers by healing my medical issues and allowing us to have one of our own, but now I truly believe you and this baby are the answer we have been patiently waiting for. I promise you, Valerie, we will love this baby with our whole hearts and *never* take for granted the sacrifice you have made."

My hands trembled as I wiped away tear after tear rolling down my cheek.

Carissa smiled and nodded, then turned to Valerie.

"This is not a decision to be taken lightly. You will probably go back and forth, changing your mind a dozen times before the baby comes, and that's O.K. If you decide to keep the baby at any point, just be very open and honest with Clair and Victor. They will not be mad at you. They care about you very much. But they deserve to know what your intentions are."

Valerie shook her head.

"I'm not changing my mind."

Carissa made arrangements to get Valerie some maternity clothes since she had just been wearing oversized shirts over unbuttoned jeans. As Valerie stood to leave, she invited us to go to her sonogram appointment at the end of the month to find out the sex of the baby.

It was mid-January yet tiny beads of sweat ran down my forehead as I watched Valerie pull out of the parking lot and drive away. I whipped around to face Carissa.

"So what do you think? Be honest."

"I think she is sincere about this. I would go ahead and start the home study and background check if I were you."

I threw my arms around her and began to cry.

"But as your friend, I will also tell you to guard your heart. Even mothers with the best of intentions can change their minds at the hospital. I don't think she realizes how hard it's going to be to hand over the baby and move on with her life, but I will do my best to prepare her for that."

Vic and I tried to contain our excitement over dinner but somehow ended up at Target®, buying gender neutral pajamas, a plethora of baby bath products and a nursery rhyme book, which I promptly hid away on a closet shelf. That way if something went awry with this whole thing I wouldn't be easily reminded.

We were somewhat taken aback when our families and friends did not share the same enthusiasm about the adoption as we did. The comments were as thoughtless as the ones I had received following my miscarriage:

"You mean you're not having a *real* baby?" I was adopted – what am *I*? A *mirage*? A *hologram*?

"*Why?*" with a look of repugnance and disdain as if we had just announced we were eating nothing but yak manure from now on.

"Well, is the mother on drugs?" *Because she would* have *to be to hand her child over to us.*

"Is she smart?" *Again, obviously* not *if she's handing her child over to us?*

"Can't you just have one of your own?" *Seriously?*

Inside, I was boiling when things like this were said to us. Valerie was an incredibly brave young woman who we had grown to love and I would not tolerate others disrespecting her in any way. This child, *our* child, was a blessing from God and would neither be treated nor talked about as a second class citizen just because I did not have the privilege of giving birth to him myself. End of discussion. Boundary lines had been drawn in the sand.

Victor and I knew we were going to have to put all emotions aside and seek the best possible legal advice we could get from someone who had our best interests at heart. We didn't have to go far. Janis Cross, our friend and partner in our firm, had an office right upstairs from us. Janis had been practicing law for thirty years, so it was no surprise that she was concerned.

"I will be happy to represent you. I *want* to. Just don't get too attached to this baby. Stay grounded and take it one day at a time," she advised, adding that she would put us on her prayer list.

It was sound advice and exactly what we would have told a client sitting on the other side of the desk. It's also so much easier said than done.

Vic ordered "What to Expect the First Year,"[11] a huge paperback book that was a tad overwhelming. It reminded me of an encyclopedia and I had no idea how I was supposed to have the entire thing read by the time the baby came with everything else that had to be done.

We needed a car seat, stroller, crib, changing table, formula, diapers, and a slew of other things. The list went on and on. Victor spent hours researching *Consumer Reports®*, narrowing down the best products and brands for our new little bundle of joy. He remained perfectly calm, at least on the outside, while I constantly seemed to be in a state of panic.

I walked into Babies 'R Us® and practically ran out in tears after ten minutes, totally and completely overwhelmed by

---

[11] Eisenberg, Arlene, Murkoff, Heidi E., and Hathaway, Sandee E. <u>What to Expect the First Year</u>. New York: Workman Publishing Company, Inc., 1989, 1996, 2008.

all the gadgets and the sheer volume of *stuff*. I didn't know what half of it was, why it was necessary, or what I was supposed to do with it. I had to resist the urge to vomit right there in the parking lot.

Valerie just laughed at us when we proudly told her about the books we had purchased and the research we had done as the three of us waited together in the lobby of her doctor's office before the sonogram. She gave us a look that clearly said what she was thinking: *amateurs*.

"You can read every book on the market, but I'm telling you it will not prepare you for everything. You're going to learn by hands-on experience. Trust me. And what works for some babies won't work for others. I have three kids and had to do things three different ways."

Valerie offered to go with us to fill out our baby registry and tell us what she found to be most helpful and what she thought was a waste of money. I was so grateful and relieved.

The nurse called Valerie's name and the three of us walked through the double doors down a long hallway. Valerie introduced us to the nurse as "the baby's parents," which warmed my heart.

"Do you want to know the sex of the baby?" the nurse asked with a smile.

All three of us nodded.

"It's a girl," Victor whispered. "I know it's a girl."

"It's a boy," I whispered back. "Valerie says it's a boy."

The nurse spread the clear gel on Valerie's growing belly and turned on the monitor. A swish-swish-swish sound broke the silence.

"That's the heart beat. Good and strong." The nurse moved the wand around in a semi-circle.

"There's the head...the spine. The hands are folded in front of the chest. There are the lungs. And there you have it – it's definitely a boy!"

I began to cry. Victor wrapped his arms around me.

"What's his name?" the nurse asked Valerie.

"Ryan Cade," she answered. "Ryan Cade Rivera."

Our precious Ryan. What a tiny little miracle. As we saw his sweet face for the first time, I closed my eyes and thanked God for this moment. This little life swimming around inside of Valerie would be our son.

"Hi, Ryan. Can't wait to meet you, little man," I said quietly.

The nurse printed out a stream of black and white pictures and handed them to Valerie, who, in turn, handed them to me.

"This is *your* baby. These are *your* pictures," she said with a smile.

My hand immediately went to my mouth to cover my quivering lip.

"Thank you so much for letting us be here today," I said as I touched her hand.

"No problem. You can come to any appointment you want to."

As we parted ways in the parking lot, Victor reached for the sonogram pictures and suggested that we go to Kinko's to make copies for our parents.

Victor was quiet on the drive there.

"Are you happy we're having a boy?" I asked, somewhat concerned.

"Yes, definitely. I'm just confused. I dreamed it was a girl."

Apparently his family was confused as well. His Aunt Jenny had felt very strongly that it was a girl, too.

"Are you *sure* Clair's not pregnant? I clearly saw a girl in my dreams," she said.

Were we sure? My emotions were totally out of whack. I was sick to my stomach a lot. Constantly exhausted. All was *not* well, that was for sure. I chalked it up to nerves and stress.

I had just been court-appointed on a very nasty family case involving allegations of sexual abuse of a child. The State was seeking termination of my client's parental rights and it was a very ugly battle that had been going on for years. As the trial setting grew near, I had spent weeks digging through boxes of discovery materials, thousands of pieces of paper that had to be examined and analyzed with precision.

I tried not to bring the pressures of work home with me, but this case refused to stay at the office. It consumed my thoughts. I thought about it when I was doing the dishes, taking a shower, and in the final moments before drifting off to sleep. Witnesses and trial strategies forced their way into my dreams. It was the biggest case I had dealt with in my short career and I saw it as a chance to not only gain some experience but to prove myself.

I found myself in tears over things I would normally consider trivial. The toilet and I were meeting face to face more often than I was comfortable with. I collapsed in bed by 8:30

p.m. every night, overcome with sheer exhaustion. I chalked it up to the upcoming trial, but there was another thought in the back of my mind as well. Although I knew chances were slim, I thought I would start eliminating the cause of this craziness by taking a pregnancy test. I had one left over from the last time I had my hopes up.

I set the test on the bathroom counter, fully expecting there to be only one pink line after the two-minute waiting period, and began getting ready for my day. In the middle of straightening a section of hair, I glanced over and did a double take. Two pink lines. *No way.* I closed my eyes, took a deep breath and shook my head. My heart began to pound and my knees felt a little shaky. *When I open my eyes, there is going to be one pink line. Ready? Open. Nope – still two.*

Victor was showering and had no idea what I was doing. It was five days away from Valentines Day. That would be a great time to tell him the news if I could wait that long. Too late. I was already pulling back the shower curtain and thrusting the test at him.

"Are you ready to be a daddy *twice* this year?"

It was a sight, really. My poor, unsuspecting husband was lathering shampoo on his head and looked like a very confused deer caught in the headlights. Maybe I should have been more specific.

"I'm pregnant."

Once again, I thrust the test at him with one hand and covered my eyes with the other, while quietly asking, "There *are* two lines, aren't there?" *Please don't tell me I'm crazy.*

At first I couldn't tell if he was happy or mad by the look on his face, but all of a sudden Victor burst out laughing and couldn't stop. He got out of the shower and, still dripping wet, gave me a big hug before getting the camera out to snap pictures of the positive pregnancy test.

Still, we were not only shell-shocked but cautious. We already had the discussion that if and when we ever got pregnant we would not tell anyone until the second trimester was safely underway. I had learned that lesson the hard way, telling people I was pregnant early on and then having to explain that I had lost the baby when they asked me weeks later how I was feeling. Talk about heart wrenching.

Now that it was a reality we could not contain our excitement. First, we decided to tell our office staff. After all, they needed to know why I was acting flakey and sick all the time. Then we thought it wasn't fair that *they* knew but our parents didn't. Then we decided that our best friends needed to know so they could be praying for this tiny being to keep growing inside of me, to hang in there. Before long, our little "secret" was no longer a secret at all. Everyone knew.

I, of course, called Jennifer the day I took the pregnancy test. She of all people knew the emotional dynamics I was struggling with. I was excited, but scared out of my mind. Overcome with fear almost to the point of being emotionally crippled.

"You can't be afraid to love this baby," Jennifer said matter-of-factly. "You have to put yourself out there and do it."

I began to sob uncontrollably.

146

"Do you think I lost the other babies because I didn't really want them? That I just wanted to make things work with Nathan? Do you think they *knew* that?"

"Honey, no. That had nothing to do with it. Stop thinking that right now."

Jennifer understood my crazy hormone surge. She was twelve weeks pregnant with their second child and had a doctor's appointment in a few days. She promised to pray for me and would call me after her appointment.

We needed all the prayer we could get. Our income was based on feast or famine. There was no stability. We had no health insurance, which wasn't such a big deal up until now since we rarely got sick. Now it would be financially devastating to pay for this pregnancy and delivery without it. Once the babies arrived, we would be bombarded with well-baby visits and shots.

Though all of this was extremely overwhelming, we were reminded that God had always taken care of us. We had never gone hungry. Bills had never gone unpaid. Even the months when we brought in very little, everything seemed to work out – not because of anything *we* had done, but because of God's provision. We knew that He would not give us these children if He did not already have a plan to provide for their needs.

I was so wrapped up in my chain of events that the email from Jennifer caught me completely off guard. She had gone to her twelve-week appointment and the doctor could not find the baby's heartbeat. A sonogram revealed that the baby had died. She was going to have a D&C in a couple of days. She did not want to talk on the phone right now but needed prayer.

I felt as though I had been hit with a soccer ball right in the gut. So this is what it feels like to have the roles reversed. I was *her* five and a half years ago. I knew the heartbreaking pain she was going through and I hated it. I sent a quick email back, telling her to call me at the office if she needed anything at all, and that I had already prayed for God to start healing her heart.

A few hours later, my receptionist was on the intercom to tell me that Jennifer was on the phone.

"Jen?"

Long pause. I could hear sniffling and a muffled cry on the other end.

"Honey, I am so sorry. What do you need from me?"

"I have to go pre-register for my...my D&C tomorrow. I can't believe this is happening to me."

I understood completely. I listened while she vented her anger and hurt, how she had to explain to her four-year-old that he wasn't going to be a big brother after all, and how his little face had twisted up before he burst into tears. He had been so excited about this baby. Everyone had.

When I heard that Jennifer's plan was to go to the hospital alone, I canceled my afternoon appointments so I could be there with her. I did not want her to be alone as I had been many years ago, with cold medical staff acting as if the loss of a precious child is just business as usual.

This time *I* was the pregnant one, trying to contain my own excitement while Jennifer was grieving. Suddenly I had a new appreciation for what she had gone through with me. It must have been really hard for her to be my friend back then. It had been all about *me*. I had never stepped away from my own

148

self-pity long enough to consider how my closest friend must have felt and for the first time I was really, really sorry.

Jennifer must have had the same revelation.

"I am so sorry you had to go through this," she said, looking down and picking at a fingernail as we waited in the hospital lobby. "I didn't know. I just...didn't know."

I reached over and grabbed Jennifer's hand. For the first time in a very long time, we understood each other. It felt as if a small piece of the invisible wall between us had been chiseled away so that we could finally look eye to eye. We knew exactly what the other was thinking without saying a single word. Old wounds that had been festering all these years finally began to heal.

****

I don't know about you, but I completely relate to Paul when he writes, "the things I don't want to do, I do. The things I *do* want to do, I don't" (Romans 7:18-19, NIV). God had revealed my stronghold of unbelief months before and had done so many amazing things since then. Still, it remained my weakness and the powers of hell could smell it a mile away.

I was on eggshells every day for the first six weeks of my pregnancy, especially after Jennifer's miscarriage. I was running to the bathroom in a panic every time I thought I felt something dripping, terrified that I was bleeding. Every little cramp sent me over the edge. I laid on the couch with my feet propped up after working all day and prayed, tears running down my face, that God would protect this baby. I was able to breathe a little easier with each passing week, knowing I had made it a little further in this pregnancy than the last.

My doctor's customary practice was to wait to see patients until they were twelve weeks along. Twelve weeks seemed like an eternity away. I was such a nervous wreck that there was no way I could make it that long without someone telling me that the baby was O.K. Fortunately, my doctor's staff was well aware of my history and agreed to see me at ten weeks.

The day before the sonogram I was a complete emotional wreck. I picked my cuticles until they bled and was feeling more nauseous than usual. Memories of my last sonogram came flooding back and I feared the worst. In the midst of the madness, I prayed a simple prayer: "Lord, I know You are here. Give me peace and calm my spirit."

Almost instantly, scripture after scripture entered my thoughts: *For God has not given us the spirit of fear; but of power, of love and of a sound mind* (2 Timothy 1:7, KJV)*; Do not be anxious about anything but in everything, by prayer and petition, with thanksgiving, make your requests known to God. And the peace of God, which transcends all understanding will guard your heart and your mind in Christ Jesus* (Philippians 4:6-7, NIV)*; Give all your worries and cares to God, for he cares about you* (1 Peter 5:7)*; There is no fear in love. True love has no room for fear because where fear is there is pain; and he who is not free from fear is not complete in love* (1 John 4:18, PEB).

I began to breathe normally as I claimed God's promises to me in His word. With each deep, calm breath, I felt all fear and worry disappear. At that moment, I knew that everything was going to be fine.

Victor and I sat in silence in the waiting room, holding hands and staring at the wall in front of us. Every so once in a while I would look at Victor and when he caught my gaze he would manage a nervous smile. I had hoped to see some sort of reassurance in his eyes, but that was more than he could offer at the moment.

I was light headed by the time we were ushered into the cold, blue sonogram room. I must have been holding my breath. I closed my eyes and began to pray as I slowly undressed. *Ok, Lord. It's show time. No matter what happens in here, I trust you. But Jesus, please let us see a living, healthy baby. Please, Father.*

God came through as promised when we heard the swish-swish-swish heartbeat on the monitor and watched the tiny gummy bear looking creature squirm ever so slightly. We were completely in awe.

"Look what you did!" the kind sonogram technician said with a smile.

The baby was only two centimeters but we knew without a doubt it was there. I was still considered "high risk" due to my history of miscarriages and damaged cervix. I needed to get as much rest as possible, stay off of my feet as much as I could, and minimize stress.

Victor and I proudly displayed the new sonogram pictures on the refrigerator next to Ryan's. Our kids. We had not yet held them in our arms, but we held them close in our hearts. We prayed for them daily. We prayed for both Valerie and me to safely carry these precious angels to full-term. We prayed for wisdom and guidance, and asked for financial blessing to meet the needs and demands of two newborns. Privately, I prayed that God would not let my heart be broken again. I pleaded with Him to not let Valerie change her mind and I begged Him to let me deliver the baby I was carrying.

The next hurdle we faced was telling Valerie that I was pregnant. We were daily bombarded with unsolicited advice on how to handle it. Most people felt we shouldn't tell her at all since she may change her mind about the adoption once she discovered we were having a baby of our own.

Vic and I never considered *not* telling Valerie. She had been so open and honest with us, even when she didn't have to be, that I felt very strongly that we owed her the same respect. We decided we would wait to tell her until I had made it through the first trimester. We had asked Valerie to go with us to register for Ryan's baby gifts and decided we would bring up the subject then, face to face.

We knew there was a possibility that everyone was right, Valerie could very well change her mind once she found out I was pregnant. The thought was absolutely terrifying. I went to God constantly with my fear, asking him to prepare Valerie's heart, give me the right words, and to calm my spirit.

Around that same time I heard a Biblical teaching about fear. The speaker defined fear in an acronym: False Evidence Appearing Real. I knew without a doubt that God had given me that teaching, as only He can do, to confirm that my fears had no bearing. I knew then and there that we were still going to be Ryan's parents.

The day came to tell Valerie and though I believed that the outcome would be good, I was still nervous. When she called

152

that morning to let us know she was not feeling well and thought she had better stay home, I had to switch to a very impromptu Plan B. My heart started pounding loudly and I felt so light headed that I half sat, half leaned against the arm of the couch as my prepared speech flew right out the window.

I took a deep breath in. "There's something we need to tell you."

Long pause. Here goes nothing.

"You're not going to believe this, but...I'm pregnant."

"You're joking."

"No, almost 13 weeks now."

"You made it! I'm so happy for you, Clair. Ryan will have a brother or sister! Wait. You're not changing your mind about the adoption, are you?"

I was so incredibly relieved to hear her say that. A huge weight lifted off my chest and I could finally breathe again.

"No! Not at all! We were afraid you might change *your* mind, but you have been so open and honest with us that we wanted to be open and honest with *you*. We have absolutely not changed our minds. We love Ryan and we want him more than anything."

Valerie started laughing.

"You are going to have your hands full. I don't envy you."

I knew she was probably right. I had no idea what it was like to have *one* newborn much less *two*. All I knew was that God would not have blessed us with these two precious babies if He was not going to equip us with the strength, love and wisdom to raise them.

153

Meanwhile, there had already been several "misunderstandings," for lack of a better word, at work. Things were not being handled the way we were told they would. Stress levels were at an all time high and things had started to get ugly. On top of that, we had no health insurance, no life insurance, no guaranteed income...and we were about to have two babies. It became abundantly clear that we were going to have to find other jobs and the sooner, the better.

Victor and I had prayed about it at great length and felt God's will was for me to be at home with the babies at least from the time Ryan was born until the end of the year. We would then see where God was leading us at that time. Our ultimate desire was for me to be able to stay home until both of them were in school. After all, they would only be little once and from what we had heard, it would go by very fast. I would have the rest of my life to work. I had wanted these precious angels so much for so long that I could not imagine handing them over to a daycare worker and missing out on all of their "firsts." I wanted to be the one to rock them to sleep, comfort them when they were scared or hurt, and instill the Christian values that were so important to us.

While we truly believed this was where God was leading us, the burden of providing for our little family fell squarely on Victor's shoulders. We wanted to stay in Amarillo more than anything, but the market for attorneys was slim to none. We weren't happy about it, but we knew we were going to have to move.

Victor had an immediate response to a resume he sent to a firm in the Dallas/Fort Worth area. It sounded promising with a steady salary which would allow me to be at home with the babies and a good benefits package, including health insurance.

I had no desire to leave the familiarity of my childhood home. Though it had once been a running joke that Amarillo is the black hole, where everyone wants so badly to leave but always ends up coming back, I had really begun to appreciate the quality of life that we had there. I loved being close to my parents, the fact that I could get anywhere in town in fifteen minutes or less, and that the local restaurants were so good that they put the big chains to shame. I loved my house, our neighbors, our church, and knowing so many people there. Yet even with all of these things, I felt complete peace about the move.

I knew without a doubt that we were placed in Amarillo, if only for a short time, for a divine purpose. If we had taken the jobs in Arizona or if I had taken the job at Potter County, decisions that made perfect sense from a human standpoint, I would never have met Valerie and we would not be getting our precious Ryan.

God's hand was so evident in the weeks leading up to Ryan's birth. We had no idea how we were going to afford all the things that a new baby needed, but we prayed and trusted God to provide. Friends began to bless us with clothes that their little boys had outgrown. Some still had the tags on them. We received piles and piles of clothes, four tubs worth, all the way from newborn to one year.

As a result of two wonderful baby showers, we brought home a closet full of diapers, enough that we did not have to buy diapers for the first four months of Ryan's life. We received our car seat, stroller, crib, bedding, bath supplies...our God met all of our needs according to his glorious riches in Christ Jesus (Philippians 4:19). He is so faithful!

We also found out that Ryan would be continued on Medicaid and was eligible for WIC until the adoption was final, so we would not have to worry about medical bills or formula for at least six months. I am still so amazed when I think about how wonderful my God is and how beautifully He provided for my sweet little boy's needs. It was as if He was saying, "You just love him. I'll take care of everything else." He always keeps His word:

> *Therefore, I tell you, do not worry about your life, what you will eat or drink; or about your body, what you will wear. Is not life more important than food, and the body more important than clothes? Look at the birds of the air; they do not sow or reap or store away in barns, and yet your heavenly Father feeds them. Are you not much more valuable than they? Who of you by worrying can add a single hour to his life?*
>
> *And why do you worry about clothes? See how the lilies of the field grow. They do not labor or spin. Yet I tell you that not even Solomon in all his splendor was dressed like one of these. If that is how God clothes the grass of the field, which is here today and tomorrow is thrown into the fire, will he not much more clothe you, O you of little faith? So do not worry, saying, 'What shall we eat?' or 'What shall we drink?' or 'What shall we wear?' For the pagans run after all these things, and your heavenly Father knows that you need them* (Matthew 6:25-32, NIV).

****

My 16 week sonogram was scheduled for May 1, 2008. We would finally find out if we were having Brooklyn Faith or Cody Ashton. Victor knew without a doubt that the baby was a girl. I had no clue. Other women would look at me with a puzzled expression and ask, "Don't you just have a *feeling*?" Unless that feeling was the constant need to pee or vomit, the answer was *no*, I had no definite feeling one way or the other. All I knew was that the baby was an active little thing that kicked even more vigorously at the sound of Victor's voice, something that made him beam with pride.

I couldn't tell if the butterflies in my stomach were from nerves or if it was the baby swimming around as the sonogram tech spread the gel on my abdomen and the image of our little miracle baby appeared on the monitor by my head. My eyes filled with tears as I saw a perfect little head, long fingers and legs like Victor and then...the "money shot." Everyone in the room saw it but me. I felt like Rachel in that *Friends* episode where she pretends like she sees her baby on the sonogram but really doesn't.

It took a few different explanations for me to see "the hamburger" as the sonogram tech so delicately put it, but it was definitely there. The tiny being inside of me was our baby girl, our Brooklyn Faith. We were ecstatic. A boy and a girl. Who could ask for more?

Children are an inheritance from the Lord. They are a reward from Him (Psalm 127:3, GW).

****

Ryan's due date was right around the corner and we had to find a place to live in Fort Worth. I was not entirely comfortable going out of town in case he came early, but I think Victor was even more anxious at the thought of choosing our home without me.

Memorial Day weekend of 2008 was a whirlwind of house hunting. Our poor realtor showed us over fifty homes in all. We made an offer on three different properties only to be outbid by other buyers. Frustrated and exhausted, we started for home early on Monday morning with another offer on the table.

We had not even left the city limits when my cell phone rang. It was Valerie's mother. I think my heart stopped.

Valerie was in the hospital and dilated to a "2." She was not progressing quickly, so it would be a while, but we would more than likely have a baby in the next 24 hours!

I watched the speedometer creep from 70 to 85 mph and said a prayer that first of all, God would forgive us for breaking the law since He usually frowns on that sort of thing; second, for our safety; third, for my bladder to hold up so we wouldn't have to stop a gazillion times for me to pee on the way home and make us get home even later; and finally, most importantly, that we would not miss Ryan's grand entrance into the world.

The phone rang again an hour later. Valerie had been sent home and there was no reason to panic or rush. Vic and I breathed a huge sigh of relief and made it back to Amarillo in the early afternoon.

A little after midnight, the phone rang again. Disoriented, Victor jumped out of bed to answer it and started rushing around to get dressed. Valerie was back in the hospital and Ryan was on his way – "for real" this time.

We grabbed pillows, a camera, and threw some things in an overnight bag. Ten minutes later we backed out of the driveway, knowing the next time we came home it would be as a family of three.

Valerie was still in labor when we reached the hospital and, considering the circumstances, was in great spirits. It was tough to watch her struggle through the pain of contractions, which were coming on fast and furious.

We had not discussed how things were going to work at the hospital with Valerie, so Victor and I had no idea what to expect. We decided to just "roll with it" and lean on the only thing we knew for sure, that God was in control.

Valerie's nurse, Wendy, ended up being a member of our church, Hillside Christian. She recognized us from a cardboard testimony[12] service two months earlier where we had stood in front of the congregation with signs that said "Struggled with having a baby" which were flipped over to read, "Adopting a son in May, and...we're pregnant!"

Wendy was excited to be a part of our answer to prayer. She pulled us aside and said that Valerie did not want to see or hold Ryan after the birth, so Wendy would immediately take him to another room to weigh and measure him. We were welcome to follow her. She also arranged for us to have a room right across from the nursery, where we could spend the next 48 hours

---

[12] To view, visit http://www.youtube.com/watch?v=RvDDc5RB6FQ. We are the very last people to go forward. To date, over 2 million people have viewed the video in its entirety.

taking care of Ryan's needs at no cost to us. We were so incredibly thankful. God is so good.

When Nurse Wendy excused herself to check Valerie's progress, Victor and I stayed in the hallway, holding each other and nervously awaiting the birth of our son. Valerie's mother stepped out, dressed in a scrub top, and said Valerie was dilated to a "10" and was about to start pushing. Valerie had sent her mom to see if I wanted to be in the room for the birth.

It was almost 2:00 a.m., but I immediately perked up as if I had downed five espressos. I quickly gave Victor a kiss, threw on a scrub top, washed my hands and awkwardly took my place by Valerie's side.

Originally deciding to do this *au naturel* as she had with her first two babies (her third had been delivered by C-section), Valerie had changed her mind at the last minute only to find out it was too late for an epidural. The whole bottom half of me was wracked with sympathy pain for her, mostly because I was overly aware of the fact that I would be in her shoes in four and a half short months. The longer I watched, the more I began to feel both faint and sick to my stomach. There was no turning back now. I would have to go through this, too. *Note to self: request epidural early on.*

Ryan Cade Rivera was born on May 27, 2008, at 2:16 a.m. Being there to welcome Ryan into the world was one of the most beautiful, amazing experiences of my life. I was absolutely overcome with emotion the very first time I laid eyes on my son. This little gray bundle with a full head of hair had made his home in my heart long before I ever saw him or held him in my arms, but seeing him for the first time only confirmed that I loved this little guy more than I ever thought possible.

Nurse Wendy wrapped Ryan in a towel, bolted through the door, and began running with him. *Why isn't he crying?* Panicked, I started running down the long corridor after her. I must have passed Victor on the way because I could hear him close behind me, asking what was wrong.

I saw Wendy duck into a room at the end of the hall and as soon as Victor and I entered, we heard the beautiful sound of Ryan's cries. Once he was placed on the cold scale, he decided to use those little lungs of his. He weighed 6 pounds 10 3/4 ounces and was 19 3/4 inches long. He had ash blonde hair and dark blue eyes. He was so tiny, so beautiful, and so perfect.

One of my favorite pictures of our new little family was taken in that room at the end of the corridor. Vic is leaning over me as I hold little Ryan, wrapped in a blanket that looked like aluminum foil with its silver insulation. We couldn't keep our eyes off of him nor the tears from falling as we thanked God over and over again for this precious baby.

I didn't want Ryan out of my sight for a single minute but Nurse Wendy convinced me that he would be just fine while she got him checked into the nursery and that if I wanted to give him his first bath, I could meet her there in about an hour.

As I watched him being rolled away in his little incubator, my thoughts immediately went to Valerie. I told Victor I would be right back and went to check on the mother of my child.

Valerie looked exhausted and rightfully so. It was now almost 3:00 a.m.

"How are you?" I sheepishly asked.

Valerie was her normal, tough-girl self.

"I'm good," she smiled. "Got an ice pack." She took a deep breath. "How is Ryan?"

My eyes welled up with tears and I wanted to tackle her with a bear hug. Keeping in mind that she was probably sore from just giving birth, I held back.

"He's beautiful. Thank you *so* much."

Her eyes began to fill with tears that she quickly blinked away.

"You are so welcome. Take good care of him, alright?"

I wiped away the hot tears that would not stop flowing with the back of my hand.

"We will. I promise you that."

"I know you will."

We sat in silence for a moment to compose ourselves. I knew Valerie wasn't comfortable with sappy emotional stuff so I quickly changed the subject and stayed with her until she was admitted to a regular room, which she had requested to be as far away from the nursery as possible. Victor and I promised to come and see her later on, and then headed for the nursery to give Ryan his first bath.

I was terrified of hurting tiny Ryan. The nurse held him under the water spout of a huge sink as I gingerly massaged soap into his hair and skin. The nurse finally took over and said, "Girl, you gotta get in there an' get all that mommy junk out," digging underneath his neck and skin folds. I had to look away. It looked like she was being so rough with him that I silently prayed, "Please don't hurt my baby!" I knew she had been doing this a lot longer than I had, and Ryan was probably not as fragile as I thought.

After the bath, Victor and I kissed Ryan goodnight, though by now it was 4:30 a.m., and collapsed in the hospital bed together, trying to get some rest. I made the nurses promise to wake us for Ryan's first feeding at 6:00 a.m. I wanted to do everything possible to bond with him, to let him know that we were his mommy and daddy, and that he was loved more than anything in this world.

For the first 24 hours of Ryan's life, Victor and I ran on pure adrenalin. We were too excited to sleep and wanted Ryan with us as much as possible. Hospital security regulations required that Ryan had to be in the nursery if we were sleeping.

One of our close friends worked at the hospital and came to visit early that morning. She brought breakfast and a door decoration that resembled a homecoming mum with a teddy bear holding a soccer ball and long, blue streamers announcing Ryan's name, date of birth and weight. We were really parents! It was the greatest feeling in the world.

Sometime in the mid-morning there was a knock at the door. It was Valerie, dressed in a hospital robe and hooked up to an IV pole.

"I was just up walking around and thought I would come and check on you."

I made a mental note to check on Valerie more while she was here. I didn't want her to think we no longer cared about her now that she had the baby. I was also suddenly aware that she could still change her mind, but I quickly determined to leave that in God's hands.

Ryan was sleeping soundly in Victor's arms.

"Do you want to see him?" I had to ask, even though I knew if she *did* it may greatly increase our chances of losing him.

Valerie stayed in the doorway and peered over at the tiny bundle in Victor's arms.

"I see him," she said, offering a weak smile.

She didn't stay much longer and we promised to visit later on.

Over the next two days we saw a lot of Valerie. Each time she inched a little closer to Ryan. She finally got close enough to take a good look at him and mentioned that he looked like his father, and although we offered, she did not want to hold him. I was secretly relieved. Although I prayed about the adoption constantly, I still struggled with a fear in the back of my mind that something could go wrong.

I hated to bring up the topic of legal paperwork with Valerie, but I had to before she was discharged from the hospital. She had to sign a release stating we could take Ryan home with us, as well as a background packet on her social, health, educational and genetic history. Our attorney's paralegal, as well as our good friend, Darla, offered to come to the hospital to notarize the preliminary forms before Valerie was released.

The voluntary relinquishment paperwork, the most important to us, could not be signed until 48 hours after Ryan's birth. Valerie would be released from the hospital by then and it would be up to her to go to our attorney's office to sign it. Valerie must have sensed my apprehension about the whole thing because more than once she reassured me that she was not changing her mind.

The last time I saw Valerie was the day she was released from the hospital. She came by our room to visit one last time and sat next to me as I snuggled the precious baby she had selflessly brought into this world. She stared at him with a sad smile on her face.

"You know, I couldn't have given him to just anybody."

I started to respond but something told me to just let her talk.

"I know that you will take good care of him. He is going to have so many things that I could never even dream of giving him. By the time I meet him, he will probably have three or four degrees like Victor and be so smart that I can't even keep up with him."

Her voice began to quiver as she stood to go.

"Tell Ryan I love him. Take care of my little one."

My eyes began to sting with tears but I managed a smile.

"We will."

Valerie turned to look at me and Ryan one last time.

"I know you will."

I said a prayer for Valerie as she walked away – for comfort, peace, and blessing. She had given us the most amazing gift and would always hold a special place in our hearts.

****

True to what everyone said, having Ryan totally changed our lives, but for the better. Even when I was a walking zombie, desperately in need of sleep and secretly mourning the days of sleeping in, I loved taking care of my little man. Every time I heard Ryan's cries on the baby monitor, no matter how exhausted I was, I remembered how long I had waited to be a mommy and how I would have gladly traded places with the new mothers who complained about the hassles of having a newborn.

That's not to say it was always easy. No one ever told me it would the hardest thing I had ever done. It was not all fluffy clouds, baby coos and sweet rosy cheeks. No one told me I would feel completely inadequate and unprepared for life with a newborn. There were times when Ryan was absolutely inconsolable. I tried everything I knew to make him stop crying but often ended up crying right along with him. I wondered why anyone ever let me leave the hospital with this precious baby when I was clearly incompetent to know how to care for him. What kind of mother doesn't know how to comfort her own baby?

I found myself on my knees a lot in those early days, asking God if He was sure I was the right woman for this. I often felt so overwhelmed with Ryan that I shuddered to think of what life would be like once Brooklyn arrived in a few short months. Each and every time, He assured me that the One who had called me was faithful and would help me (I Thessalonians 5:24), and that I could do all things through Him who strengthens me (Philippians 4:13).

****

It was early October yet there were no recognizable signs of fall in the Dallas/Fort Worth area. I had grown accustomed to putting away all summer clothes by mid-September and breathing in the unmistakable crispness in the air, a mixture of fallen leaves and cooler temperatures that I found intoxicating. It was something I looked forward to each year. Who would have thought that a mere five hours away from home it could be so very different?

In the spirit of festivity, I had picked up a bright orange shirt at Motherhood Maternity and now, nine months pregnant, very much resembled a large pumpkin. With my due date rapidly approaching, my best friend, Kelly, and I had splurged on pedicures and had pumpkins painted on our big toes. At least I blended in with the fall decorations.

Donned in the pumpkin shirt, I headed to my 39 week appointment. For the most part, the pregnancy had gone smoothly. At 28 weeks, I had gone to the emergency room with severe lower back pain. My doctor put me on medication and bed rest to prevent pre-term labor, and things had been fine ever since. As blessed as I felt to have made it this far, I was growing more and more uncomfortable.

Nervousness and excitement set in as I sprawled awkwardly on the examining table, my bottom half covered only by a big, glorified napkin (why bother, really?) that seemed to grow shorter every visit, and it ripped when I attempted to wrap it around me. At the last appointment, my doctor had mentioned induction as a possibility and I was absolutely positive that she would schedule one today.

No such luck. I was barely dilated and Brooklyn had not dropped enough to justify an induction. I was told it could be another week, maybe even two or three. Not exactly what I wanted to hear. I waddled down the hall, shoulders hunched in defeat, to schedule an appointment for the following week.

I called Victor as soon as I got in the car to let him know there was no need to schedule any days off for an induction. Next, I called my mother-in-law, Gladys, who had taken Ryan to her mother's, to let her know Brooklyn was apparently quite comfortable where she was at and not coming any time soon.

Gladys reminded me that when she was pregnant with Victor, she had fallen asleep and woke up drenched. She actually thought she had wet the bed, but it turned out her water had broken. She had no pain, no noticeable contractions, but went to the hospital anyway just to make sure everything was alright. She was shocked to find out she was already dilated and it was time to have a baby.

"It will happen soon. Don't worry. Get some rest, and I will bring Ryan home in an hour or so," she said.

My last phone call was to my parents. By this time, the pregnancy hormones had washed over me like a tide on the seashore and I was close to tears. My mom (Darlene) told me the same thing that Gladys had, that Brooklyn would be here soon enough and to go lay down before Ryan came home.

My pillow was wet with tears when I drifted off to sleep, praying that God would bring this baby safely into the world in *His* timing, not mine, and to give me the strength and patience I needed to get through the rest of this pregnancy.

A strange sensation woke me about an hour later. I felt a warm liquid coming out of me and wondered the same thing that Gladys had – if I had wet the bed. Startled, I jumped up to head to the bathroom and as soon as I stood up I felt a gush of fluid run down my legs onto the floor.

I shuffled to the bathroom, walking bowlegged, and stood over a towel as I dialed my doctor's office.

"Yes, I just left there a couple of hours ago and was told I was nowhere *near* having this baby, but I have a lot of fluid coming out of me..."

After a series of questions, the nurse determined that my water broke, which is what I figured this mess was even though I had no pain or contractions, and to head to the hospital. My heart began to spin as I grabbed the overnight bag and began packing all the last minute stuff while balancing the phone on my shoulder to call Victor, who assured me he would be right there. Then I called Gladys.

"You know that thing that happened to you when you were having Victor? It just happened to me, exactly the way you described."

It was rush hour, which meant it took Victor about an hour to get home and another hour or so to get to Baylor All-Saints Hospital in downtown Fort Worth. I finally started having contractions on the way to the hospital. Victor scrawled the times down on a napkin as we sat stalled in traffic, but they were short, sporadic, and really not that painful.

A calming peace settled over me once we got to the hospital. I was no longer scared, no longer nervous. Though I had no idea what to expect, I focused on what I *did* know. I knew God promised to never leave me or forsake me (Hebrews 13:5) and that he was with me always (Matthew 28:20). Together, we would get through this.

Brooklyn Faith Rivera was born at 2:06 a.m. on October 8, 2008, eight hours after we were admitted to the hospital. She weighed 7 pounds, 8 ounces, and was 19 inches long. She had a head full of dark hair and the most beautiful, bright eyes I had ever seen.

I was so relieved that Brooklyn was finally here and that she was perfect in every way. I was instantly full of overwhelming love and admiration for this tiny creature I had nurtured for nine months. I wanted her with me as much as possible and found myself just staring at her in amazement. She was so incredibly beautiful and I had never felt more blessed in all my life.

The night we brought Brooklyn home from the hospital, Victor and I were sitting on the couch with both babies and we suddenly looked at each other like, "How did *this* happen?" In a matter of a few months, we had gone from being a *couple* to a family of *four*. It was very humbling to recognize this as not only a huge responsibility but a monumental blessing from God. He had chosen *us* to parent these two precious little ones.

It was definitely an adjustment, getting into a routine with two newborns to look after. I was on my own for a majority of the day with our little bundles of joy, and while I loved every minute of it, I had never been more overwhelmed or exhausted from a job in my life. I was on the go non-stop from the time I got up until my head hit the pillow.

Slightly offended by an off-hand comment (from someone who had *obviously* never stayed home with children) that it must be so nice to have so much "free time" and when was I "going back to work?" as if I were lying around by a sparkling pool with cucumbers on my eyes, having a cabana boy bring me drinks with paper umbrellas in them. I made a concerted effort to record the events of one day in a journal to vindicate myself from such thoughtless scrutiny...

Having just drifted off into a deep slumber after the 3:00 a.m. feeding, my head darts up from my pillow, drool string attached, when I hear my two month old, Brooklyn, crying again. I glance at the alarm clock. 6:50 a.m. Rise and shine time. I stumble out of bed and trudge to the kitchen to put a bottle in the warmer, then return to my screaming daughter to change her diaper, something to pass the time until her bottle is ready. Once she is fed and burped, she drifts back off to sleep. Ah, the sweet sound of silence. I crawl back into bed and snuggle under the covers.

Exactly five seconds later I hear my six month old, Ryan, crying. Same routine begins again. I get out of bed, put a bottle in the warmer, change his diaper and set him on the floor in his Boppy® pillow where he feeds himself while watching PBS. I run into the bedroom and pull my hair back in a ponytail. I then wash and sterilize bottles for the first of many times today and get my husband's lunch together, trying to fit in sips of coffee between tasks.

While I'm burping Ryan, I hear Brooklyn crying in the next room. I feel something moist. Spit up on my right shoulder - a tried and true badge of motherhood. Only it's also on my pants.

No time for changing clothes, though. I dab at it with the burp rag and go to Brooklyn's room.

By the time I get to her she's in full fledged fit throwing. I change her diaper and get back to the living room only to find that Ryan has spit up on my hardwood floor. I plead with him to be still while I find a safe place to set Brooklyn down. Too late. He rolls over into the spit up. I scoop him up and take him to his room to change his clothes. Brooklyn screams the whole time.

I get Ryan cleaned up and return to the living room to a highly offensive smell. Brooklyn, still screaming, has a dirty diaper so rank that I think the paint is starting to peel. I set Ryan down on the floor to play, scoop up Brooklyn, change her diaper and return to the living room to find that Ryan has spit up yet again and is smearing it with his hands.

I put Brooklyn in the swing, pick up Ryan, change his clothes, wash his hands and face and return to the living room. Brooklyn is asleep. Ryan plays quietly while I start a load of laundry and clean up breakfast dishes. I look over at Ryan to see how he's doing and I see "the face" that every mother knows and loves: the one that says "I'm cooking up something special for you in the diaper department." I wait until the face subsides then change his diaper.

In the midst of this I realize I have been up for three hours and have not yet gone to the bathroom or eaten and I need to do both...badly. Before the thought has even finished processing, Brooklyn is crying again. It's time to feed her. Ryan is crying, too. It's time for his nap. I put a bottle in the warmer for Brooklyn and put Ryan to bed.

I read my Bible while feeding Brooklyn. She falls asleep after her feeding and I quickly email my husband a devotional, insight from my daily reading. I hit send and hear Ryan waking up from his nap. It's time for him to eat.

I mix cereal and baby food and launch into the daunting task of getting the rice and carrots into Ryan's mouth and having it *stay* there rather than end up in his hair, on the table, on the floor, and all over me.

I look at the clock, realize it's 12:15 p.m. and I still have not peed or eaten. I put Brooklyn in the bouncy seat and quickly run to the bathroom, shoving a piece of lunch meat rolled up in a slice of cheese in my mouth. I catch a glimpse of myself in the bathroom mirror. *Oh noooo...*not good. Not only do I look like a bag lady in my oversized sweats, no makeup and messy ponytail...not only do I look incredibly tired...I have dried spit up, snot, and carrots on my shirt. It was 180 degrees from my previous life of business suits, carefully styled hair, and full makeup. Who *is* this woman staring back at me? Not only do I not recognize her, but I'm a little afraid of her!

With the afternoon in full swing, there is much left to be done. But wait - it's time for Brooklyn to eat again. She's reminding me by screaming at the top of her lungs. The neighbors probably think I'm beating her. Child Protective Services has surely been on speed dial for months now. Ryan joins in, letting me know he is bored of being in the jumpy jump.

I move Ryan to the swing and put in an Elmo video, plopping next to him in the glider with Brooklyn and bottle in hand. Ryan takes one look at the bottle, and the fact that I'm holding someone other than him, and screams. I talk softly to him, smile, and try to get him to look at Elmo but he continues to scream of my betrayal. This continues for seven full minutes (yes, I'm counting) until he nods off in mid-scream. I finish feeding Brooklyn and put her down for a nap as well.

Ah – silence. I crawl into bed, close my eyes and start to doze off when Ryan begins to cry. I put him on his play mat with some toys and think about popping in an exercise video when I realize that four loads of laundry have piled up and need to be folded. *Note to self: carrots stain.*

In the midst of folding, I look over at Ryan and see that he has spit up more carrots on the floor, on his clothes, the Exersaucer...anything within a three foot radius and he's rolled in it so it's in his hair as well. I give him a bath, glance at the clock, and realize it's time to start dinner. Brooklyn begins to fuss, so I pick her up and gently rock her to sleep. She's dead to the world until the moment I set her down in her crib. Weeping and gnashing of teeth begin. Guilt sets in and I feel like the worst mom in the world for letting her cry. Meanwhile, Ryan starts wailing. As long as I'm holding him he's fine. The minute I try to set him down he screams. I determine he's still tired and put him in his crib, moving onward to the kitchen.

As I start getting everything out of the cupboards and cabinets, the phone rings and I breathe a sigh of relief to see on the caller ID that it's Victor. Awesome. I balance the phone on my shoulder, stir dinner and unload the dishwasher. I am the multi-task queen. Dinner is in the oven. Ryan is fussy again and wants me to jump up and down and/or dance.

Knowing my husband is about to walk in the door, I take one more look in the mirror and realize I'm still in my pajamas from this morning. It's 6:25 p.m. *What the heck?* I throw on some clothes while both babies cry in the next room. Being out of their sight – even momentarily - is now a misdemeanor offense punishable by enduring incessant crying and/or wailing.

I wash the pots and pans used to make dinner and make more bottles rather than put on makeup, calm a screaming Ryan and feed a hungry Brooklyn. Victor walks in the door so I get dinner served while he entertains the babies. After washing dinner dishes, I prepare Vic's lunch for the next day and set the coffee pot to turn on at 6:15 a.m. Vic and I give both kids a bath (Ryan now holds the record for "most spit ups in a twelve hour period"), get their pajamas on, read a story, give Ryan a bottle and put him to bed at 10:00 p.m.

Exhausted, I announce I'm taking a bath and try my hardest to relax while Brooklyn cries in the background. Not sure what's going on, I cut my bath short and come into the living room to find my husband trying to calm her down. She's hungry *now* and a bottle is still warming. We sit through five minutes that feels like fifteen hours of intense screaming, get her fed and put her to bed.

We read our devotional for couples and I crawl into bed. It's 11:46 p.m. I thank God for the miracle of these two precious little lives that He's entrusted me with and also pray that Brooklyn will sleep at least 4 hours. I drift off to sleep until the baby monitor wakes me at 4:40 a.m. Yes! We made it 5 hours. Time to start another day...

So much for "free time!" But you know what? I love every crazy minute of my life. I start off each day by praying for God to love my children through me, to give me His strength and wisdom, and to accomplish His purpose in me that day. Life was still a three-ring circus that first year with the babies; however, God's grace not only got me through it, but helped me to relax and enjoy those precious moments. He gave *this* childless woman a family, making her one happy mother! Praise the Lord! (Psalm 113:9).

Becoming a mother has taught me so much about many things, but none more than the nature of God. I finally began to grasp His love for me as His child as my love for my own children began to unfold. I love them so unconditionally.

There are times I just cannot keep my eyes off of Ryan. I am overcome with love for him and I often scoop him up, kiss his sweet little face and tell him what a precious gift he is to us. I often stare at Brooklyn, my little miracle baby, in amazement. When she looks up at me with her daddy's eyes, it takes my breath away. The little girl that we were told would never be is right here in my arms. I am often overcome to the point of tears and in these moments all I can do is whisper, "thank you, Jesus."

It is times like this, times of complete gratitude, when I sometimes feel God speaking to me in a new and profound way. One precious time in particular comes to mind. Brooklyn had fallen asleep in my arms and I was overcome with love for her. As I stroked her face with my finger, I felt God speak to my spirit. *"Do you know that I look at you with the very same kind of admiration, amazement, and love? I love you so much, my child, that I want to draw you close to me each and every day, and tell you how precious you are to me. I am so glad that you are mine."*

I realized that I had never fully accepted the depth of His love for me. He loves me and delights in me simply because I am His child, just like I love and delight in my "little man" and my "tiny girl" because they are *mine*.

Another such moment happened when Ryan was about seven months old. Vic and I were beginning to get concerned because he was not crawling yet. Oh, he got around. He could roll. He could pivot around on his tummy. He could crawl backward. He *wanted* to move forward and got so frustrated when he couldn't reach something or go somewhere he wanted to go. I tried to show him by helping him move his arms and knees forward. Victor tried to show him by demonstrating (and we really should have videotaped that).

There were times when Ryan was so close to crawling. The joy of anticipation filled my heart as I got down on the floor about a foot away from the little guy, who had pulled himself up on his hands. I held my hands open, gave him a big smile of encouragement and encouraged him to "come to Mommy," but he was tired and frustrated. He did not want to come to me. He wanted me to pick him up and move him to where he wanted to go. And honestly, it hurt so much to watch him struggle that everything in me wanted to do just *that*. But because I love Ryan with all of my heart, I wanted him to grow and go through all the stages he needed to go through, no matter how painful it would be for both of us. If I continued to do everything for him, I would end up crippling him in a multitude of ways.

In that moment, God spoke to my heart. *"I know exactly how you feel, child. There were so many times in your life that I just wanted you to come to me, to take that first step toward deliverance from whatever you were struggling with at the time. Now do you see why I had to let you go through some of those things? You needed to grow. Do you see how painful it was to be so close to you, watching you cry out to me and wonder why I wasn't doing anything to alleviate your pain?"*

Another time, I was studying the book of Psalms and I came across a verse that says *Keep me as the apple of your eye* (Psalm 17:8, NIV). I had to stop and read it again. I sang to Brooklyn every night, a song I had made up just for her. One of the lines was that she was the apple of our eye. It was as if God was letting me know, in a very personal way, that He delights in me as much as I delight in Brooklyn.

Time after time, He has revealed the depth of His love for me through seemingly insignificant moments with my children. These moments have brought me tremendous healing and freedom in Christ. It is a love far greater than I have ever known or experienced, deeper than I had ever thought possible.

****

On December 12, 2008, we stood as a family in front of Judge James Anderson in the Randall County Court at Law #1. Dressed in a three-piece suit just like his daddy, Ryan officially became our son. It was as if I had been holding my breath, waiting to exhale, for six months. Now, like a deflating balloon, I could slowly, steadily, breathe out and relax. No one could take Ryan away from us now.

Tuning out the laughter and chatter of family, friends, and on-lookers, I slowly scanned the room and let the impact of what had just happened sink in. My dad, quietly taking pictures from the corner of the courtroom, had the glistening of tears in his eyes. Thirty-three years ago he had been in my shoes, making the same promises under oath and probably feeling the same sense of relief to finally, officially be a parent to a baby he had already come to love as his own.

Victor held Ryan on his hip and beamed with pride as a small crowd gathered around to congratulate us and meet our little man. Among them were Cindy Gilliland and Carissa Wingate, our dear friends at Special Delivery, who had been by our sides from the very beginning of this adoption adventure. Janis Cross, our attorney who had become not only our mentor but close friend, smiled and cooed at Ryan, who held his little arms out for her to hold him. I glanced down in my arms at sweet baby Brooklyn, so stunningly beautiful in her red velvet dress and matching headband with a bow that was bigger than her head. I marveled at this little wonder as she yawned and stretched in my arms.

As I took in all of these things, I knew without question that I was blessed beyond measure. I can finally say with confidence that God never wastes a hurt. It had been a long and rocky path with many unplanned pit stops and detours, but it had led me here. My little family was worth the heartache and worth every loss. And to think of all the times I questioned God's methods and timing.

> *I know that you can do all things; no plan of yours can be thwarted. You asked, 'Who is this that obscures my counsel without knowledge?' Surely I spoke of things I did not understand, things too wonderful for me to know...My ears had heard of you but now my eyes have seen you...*
>
> *[T]he Lord made him prosperous again and gave him **twice as much** as he had before... The Lord blessed the latter part of Job's life more than the first* (Job 42:2-3, 5, 10, 12, NIV, emphasis mine).

Twice as much. Every time I read this, chills run down my spine. To think I had avoided the Book of Job like the plague when I was hurting so much, scoffing at the suggestion that I read it in the midst of my pain. God had now used this very same book to show me not only His sovereignty over my circumstances but to shower me with blessings. I had gone from no children to having two – twice as much as I had before – all because I had finally surrendered my own desires in exchange for God's amazing plan for my life.

I am so humbled that God would choose me, *entrust* me to be these precious babies' mother with all of my imperfections, weaknesses, past failures, and insecurities. More than once I have come to God the way Moses did to ask if He is sure He has the right person for this great responsibility. Each and every time He reminds me that His grace is sufficient and His strength is made perfect in my weakness (2 Corinthians 12:9).

I am reminded of our friend Hannah each and every day. The words she spoke when she brought Samuel, the son she had longed for, to the temple to present him to the Lord have such a special meaning to me. They were once displayed on a plaque in the entryway of my parents' house underneath a portrait Mary

Ann had painted of me before she died. A framed copy now hangs in each of my children's rooms, a gift from my birthmother, Rachel:

For this child I prayed and the Lord has granted my request.
As long as [s]he lives [s]he belongs to Him
(1 Samuel 1:27-28, NKJV).

Epilogue

"Twins?" the cashier asked as I maneuvered the double stroller through the checkout line.

Brooklyn, now nine months old, had one foot propped up on the stroller and the other in her mouth. Thirteen-month-old Ryan sat quietly behind her, eating cereal puffs.

"Actually, no. They're four months apart."

The cashier's smile soon began to fade as she arched her eyebrows.

"Are they both *yours*?"

"Yes," I nodded while putting the rest of my groceries on the conveyor belt.

"So one is adopted, right?"

I took a deep breath. Avoiding sarcastic comments was quickly becoming a new personal challenge for me.

"Yes."

"Which one?" She glanced first at Brooklyn, then at Ryan.

I honestly had to stop and think about it. Both of them are sewn into the fabric of my heart in such a way that I don't even think about the fact that I didn't give birth to both of them anymore. This revelation made me smile as I turned to her and said, "I don't remember."

www.ingramcontent.com/pod-product-compliance
Lightning Source LLC
Chambersburg PA
CBHW021100090426
42738CB00006B/432